THE MODERN
TROPHY
WIFE

THE MODERN
TROPHY
WIFE

How to Achieve Your *Life Goals* While Thriving at Home

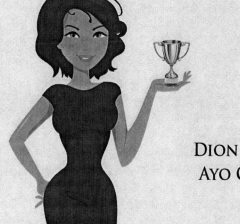

DION METZGER, MD
AYO GATHING, MD

The Modern Trophy Wife: How to Achieve Your Life Goals While Thriving at Home

A Modern Trophy Life Series Book

This book is not intended as a substitute for the medical or psychiatric advice of a personal physician. The reader should regularly consult a physician in matters relating to his or her health and particularly with respect to any symptoms that may require diagnosis, counseling, or medical attention. Any use of the information in this book is at the reader's discretion.

Cover design and artwork: Suzana Stankovic

Book design: Michael Rehder

ISBN 978-0-9977281-1-8 (paperback)
ISBN 978-0-9977281-2-5 (hardcover)
eISBN 978-0-9977281-0-1

Library of Congress Control Number: 2016913486

Published in Atlanta, GA. Printed in the United States of America

16 17 18 0 9 8 7 6 5 4 3 2 1

To our mothers,
Sheila Flemming-Hunter, PhD and
Clevelette Austin, MBA, CMA.
These two women are the ultimate
Modern Trophy Wives.

Contents

INTRODUCTION... XI

MEET THE AUTHORS XV

CHAPTER 1:
THE MODERN TROPHY WIFE LOVES HERSELF...........1
Refuel Your Own Tank 2
Make Sleep a Priority: Wind Down Before You Fall Down............. 4
Exercise: Medicine for the Body and Mind 5
The Power of Confidence.. 7

CHAPTER 2:
THE MODERN TROPHY WIFE HAS LIFE GOALS........ 13
Healthier Habits 13
Your Inner Circle 14
The MTW Protocol: Dream, Believe, Do........................ 15

CHAPTER 3:
THE MODERN TROPHY WIFE BALANCES ROLES....... 25
Be in the Moment.. 26
Wifey vs. Mommy.. 29
Balancing Tips for Wifey and Mommy 31

CHAPTER 4: THE MODERN TROPHY WIFE
MAKES HER OWN RULES 41
Self-Awareness 42
Identify What Fulfills You 44
What Does Your Success Look Like?............................ 46
Stop Comparing Yourself to Others............................ 46
Do More of What You Love 48
Focus on the Positive... 49

CHAPTER 5: THE MODERN TROPHY WIFE MANAGES TIME EFFECTIVELY 55

The Pitfalls of Overscheduling 55
Tips to Get More out of Your Time................................58
Fight Procrastination 61
Better Time Management = Better You.........................64

CHAPTER 6: THE MODERN TROPHY WIFE BUILDS STRONG RELATIONSHIPS 69

Teamwork Makes the Dream Work 70
#SquadGoals...72
The Golden Rule..76
Male Supports 77
It Takes a Village 79

CHAPTER 7: THE MODERN TROPHY WIFE IS A ROLE MODEL AND MENTOR 83

The Mentor-Mentee Relationship..............................84
Are You Role Model or Mentor Material?.........................86
Your Child Is Watching 90
Pay It Forward 93
The Modern Trophy Wife Hall of Fame 95

CHAPTER 8: THE MODERN TROPHY WIFE IS WILLING TO STEP OUT OF HER COMFORT ZONE..99

Go for the "New"...99
Vertical Career Moves...101
Travel, Meet, and Grow...104
Overcome the Fear...105

CHAPTER 9: THE MODERN TROPHY WIFE IS A SECURE WOMAN 111

Independence vs. Interdependence vs. Codependence.............112

Healthy Boundaries: Ready, Set, Maintain! 114

CHAPTER 10: THE MODERN TROPHY WIFE IS EMPOWERED IN RELATIONSHIPS.................... 123

The Marriage Shift..124

The Effects on Relationships of Marrying Later 126

Fertility Matters 131

Let's Talk About Sex 133

CONCLUSION 139

BONUS CHAPTER: THE MODERN TROPHY WIFE STARTED AS A TROPHY WOMAN 143

Enjoy Your Single Experience 144

Dating with Deal-Breakers 146

ENDNOTES 151

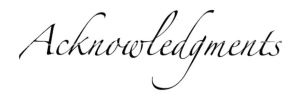

Acknowledgments

We would like to express our gratitude to the many people who saw us through this process and helped us bring this book to life. We acknowledge all those who provided inspiration and support, offered comments, and assisted in the editing, proofreading, and design.

First, we would like to thank our manager, mentor, and friend Ms. Lise Richards. Without you, this book never would have seen the light of day.

We would like to thank Mrs. Christina Roth for her guidance and expertise during proofreading and editing.

Thank you to Mr. Michael Rehder for the amazing illustration and design.

Thank you to Dr. Robby Short for giving life and a wealth of knowledge that we can now share with the world.

Thank you to Mrs. Alero Afejuku, Esq. and Mrs. Carol Green von Kaul, Esq. for your assistance and sound legal contributions.

Thank you to Mr. Ken Austin for your belief in our concept and sharp eye during pre-editing.

Thank you to Mr. Robert Hunter for your ongoing support in our endeavors.

Thank you to our trusted friends for your encouragement and continued dedication over the years.

Last but not least, we want to thank our husbands, Aziz Metzger and Jason Gathing. Without your love, care, and patience, we could not be the Modern Trophy Wives that we strive to be.

Introduction

We are sure you have seen her. Sitting at the stoplight, pumping her gas, or walking down the aisle of a grocery store. She seems to do everyday things with an aura of assurance, so you can't help but look at her a second longer. She seems to have it all together. She's beautiful but doesn't scream "watch me!" She's stylish but doesn't necessarily sport designer duds. She's smart but not a know-it-all. She's the kind of woman who would seemingly intimidate other females and daunt male suitors, but instead she inspires awe. You wonder what it's like to be her or to be with her. Even more amazing, she doesn't brag about her magnificence. She is humble and authentic, the first to admit that in spite of all of her successes, she has faults and has had failures. This well-rounded and smart woman is becoming an aspiration in the twenty-first century. A sex symbol, even.

This new ideal of woman is a stark contrast from the traditional notion of feminine appeal. She is what we have termed "the Modern Trophy Wife." The Modern Trophy Wife is a confident and well-balanced woman who seeks to enrich herself and the world around her. She embodies femininity and empowers others while achieving her dreams. When she arrives on her man's arm, everyone notices—he must be smart for choosing a woman like her!

We've seen glimpses of her in the past. Jackie Kennedy. Princess Diana. Coretta Scott King. But now, she is seen more frequently and is more visible in various industries. Michelle Obama. Amal Clooney. Priscilla Chan. Beyoncé. They are icons in their own right, a symbol of the turning tide in big-city USA as well as small-town America. Men are yearning for a new type of woman. A woman who can be his complement, not his competition. A woman who stimulates his mind, not just his body. A woman who can hold her own in the boardroom and the bedroom. The Modern Trophy Wife is that and so much more.

THE MODERN VS. TRADITIONAL TROPHY WIFE

The phrase *trophy wife* has baggage and preconceived notions. From ancient Egyptian goddesses to new millennium supermodels, civilizations have marveled at women primarily for their beauty. History has well documented its fascination with gorgeous women; hell, a mythological war was initiated over Helen's feminine wiles! There the women were, etched in stone, smiling on a billboard, or walking down a runway. But the most common image of all has been the trophy wife standing on the arm of some immensely wealthy man.

Affluent men often make a statement regarding their status by presenting a strikingly beautiful companion at their sides. CEOs showcase their stunning mates. Kings parade their queens. Admirers look on in wonder; others with disdain. The traditional trophy wife, usually the second wife, doesn't say much as her role is to be seen, not heard. Everyone knows not to ask too many questions about her, but if they dared, the facts were never memorable. *How old is she?* Young . . . and the younger, the better! *What does she do?* Exfoliate! *What are her goals?* To be a wife! And quite often, she becomes just that.

Yes. That beauty typically had her eyes on the altar—on a life of influence and wealth—while her man was still married. She was not present in the building stages of the empire but looked every bit an empress. The often-present first wife may no longer have looked the part when her love and support finally paid off for her man. She was no longer deemed fit for his evolving story; and this is where the next chapter began: the era of the traditional trophy wife.

The traditional trophy wife was often the second or third wife, who charmed the pants right off her man after he made it to the top. She was not just a mate but also a symbol to the world that he was rich and powerful. Now he could have not only any possession he wanted, but any *one* that he wanted. And she was a sight to see. She could easily have been mistaken for a runway model or beauty queen. However, she may not have been able to succeed on the talent or Q & A portion of the competition! She was rarely an intellectual or academic match for her well-to-do husband. But money was their connection, not interests or intellect. Both parties enjoyed it, wanted more of it, and did what it took to get it. Rinse, wash, and repeat.

No doubt some men are still destined to fall for a woman with the face of an angel and the body of a goddess, but no brains to boot. These fellows are as excited as a kid in a candy store as they wade through a sea of gorgeous women, with their eyes on the prize of hooking an amazing catch. But in recent years, there has been a shift in this age-old tale, tweaks in the narrative. The storybook Princess began to have ideas to help her Prince become a great King. First Ladies began to have their own political agendas. Television moms started having careers. Slowly but surely, the prized wife evolved into the epitome of brains and class. The wealthy man now stands next to a bombshell with a more polished look. A woman who shines brighter than the traditional trophy wife who came before her. She just has "it." That "it" factor. She is a Modern Trophy Wife, and she owns it.

THE MODERN TROPHY WIFE MISSION

This work is not an instructional guide on how to impress a man or become a wife. This book is about how to do what people say we as women can't: have it all! Traditional Western culture assumes that a woman cannot succeed at being a loving mate, as a nurturing parent, and in her profession. Fear and guilt have been drilled into our subconscious, so we are hesitant to even dream of having it all. We want that promotion, but are scared of neglecting our family. We want that second child, but we're fearful of what our bosses will think. Even a desire to take a "me day" feels selfish. Ladies, we're here to tell you to release that fear, worry, and guilt. Your trajectory should be decided by you, not by those around you. It's time to allow yourself to dream the impossible. Set goals that appear unattainable. Aspire to be the best!

The Modern Trophy Wife will take you through the character, mindset, and routine of the woman who dares to want more and gets it. Whether you are a young woman new to dating or to the workforce or are married with children in a career or relationship rut, this book is for you. It will show you how to approach life and navigate daily situations to flourish in all settings. We will teach you how to think, act, and behave in order to progress in every area of your life. After reading this book, you will learn how to reach your goals while thriving at home, and do it with style.

We wrote this book because we have been where you are. We weren't always balanced, confident women with husbands and families. Not even close! We were once just two young women looking for love, chasing our dreams, and trying to enjoy ourselves along the way. Throughout our lives we learned valuable lessons, many from one another, and we want to share them with you. We want to help you get where you've pictured yourself in your wildest imagination. We are going to talk real with you, like we do with each other during our ladies' night out dinners. We are going to be informative yet open, unfiltered, and empowering. You are one of us now; one of the girls. Welcome to the Modern Trophy Wife inner circle.

Meet the Authors

As you work your way through *The Modern Trophy Wife*, you'll notice an author stamp at the beginning of each chapter. That stamp indicates which of us has written that particular chapter. This approach allows us to contribute our unique perspectives, both personally and professionally, to a specific topic. This means you get the best of both worlds to become the best Modern Trophy Wife possible!

Now, we will introduce each other to give you a glimpse of who we are and how our friendship began!

MEET DR. METZGER

I have known Dion since we were seventeen years old. Where did the time go?! From adolescent coeds to practicing physicians, we have literally grown up together personally and professionally. On the outside looking in, one might think that she and I are very similar. We are women who are close in age, completed our medical training at the same institutions, and chose psychiatry as a specialty. Not to mention we are both extroverted, family oriented, and major foodies!

But when you take a closer look at our lives and experiences, there are major differences that have influenced our views and perspectives on the world. I was raised in a single-parent home in the South; Dion grew up in a two-parent home in the Northeast. My family was lower middle class as my mother was an educator at a small, historically black college, while Dion grew up more affluent as the child of a physician and an accountant. I had an older sister and was the baby of the family, whereas Dion was the elder of two.

These differences didn't matter; we used them to learn from one another. Many of the lessons I have absorbed from her over time have been unspoken. You don't always think about how much your friends influence you or broaden your horizons, but I know for sure that Dion has done it in a positive way for me. This near two decades of friendship not only influenced me, but some of what I learned from Dion also gave me ideas for this book, some essentials of a Modern Trophy Wife.

A woman should have clear standards and deal-breakers

I'll never forget a conversation that Dion and I had years ago. At that time, we were both single and dating, so we had been experiencing a number of interesting characters. She had met a man who we both thought was promising, so I was surprised to learn that she was ending things. When I asked her about it, she said plainly, "He never takes me out; he tries to beer and DVD me." And that was the end of him! She learned how men should treat women, and as a result, she would not compromise her ideals. She learned that she has worth and was therefore unwilling to settle for someone who would not recognize her value. A man who would not court her was a deal-breaker, and anyone not living up to her expectations was not worth her time.

However, these standards pertained not only to dating. Dion has standards for anyone wanting to be in her life. This includes relatives, friends, and colleagues. No one takes advantage of her or repeatedly lets her down. Dion always demands respect!

It is not weak to be vulnerable

One thing I admire about Dion is that she believes in love. She always knew there was someone out there for her, and if she continued to have faith, they would find each other. I once compared her to J. Lo, a self-proclaimed romantic who loves being in love. In order to begin the journey to a happy ending, Dion was willing to let her guard down. This was difficult for me! I saw mostly broken relationships growing up, so I was reluctant to open up to someone who could hurt me. I often laugh to myself when thinking about our younger days; I thought Dion was crazy for continuing to look for love after heartbreak. She once said, "What's the worst that can happen? If I get my heart broken, I'm not going to die. It may feel like it, but I won't." So true!

I eventually realized that being vulnerable and trusting someone makes you strong, not weak. Putting up walls helps to protect you from being hurt, but it also blocks out the blessings and positive things. Keeping an open mind and allowing yourself to receive and give love is one of the most beautiful things in the world; and while it is not always perfect, it has certainly paid off for both of us.

You can be a cool mom

Until the last few years, I had never really thought about what kind of mother I would be. I love children and work with them daily, but I never pictured myself in that role. So when I found out that Dion was going to be a mother, I couldn't wait to see how that process would affect her.

I'll never forget the first time I visited Dion after she had her first child. She opened the door dressed in a fashionable outfit with her hair and nails on point. I remember forgetting for a split second that I had come to visit her to see the new baby. She exuded an aura of ease and naturally held her infant while discussing her plans for the next few months. She intended to research tasks to promote her new son's development, get herself into stellar physical shape, and eventually transition back to work. She also mentioned that in the next couple of months we needed to get our girls' night out events back on the calendar. I was in awe of her collectivity. She was still every bit of the relaxed, easygoing friend I knew and loved. She hadn't changed a bit! And at that very moment I was inspired; I could also be a mom, and a cool one at that.

MEET DR. GATHING

Ayo and I arrived in Atlanta, Georgia, in 1998. As bright-eyed teenagers, we moved from opposite ends of the country into our freshman dorms on different college campuses. We had no idea our paths would soon intertwine into decades of friendship. We met through a mutual friend at a party. We quickly noticed we had similar dreams, including our desire to become doctors. Our friendship bloomed at lightning pace. We went on to share many milestones together—from accepting medical school scholarships to entering the same psychiatry residency program to toting our plastic veils at each other's bachelorette parties. She is brilliant, kind, and fun—the embodiment of a Modern Trophy Wife.

Brilliant

If I were on a game show and had to call a friend, Ayo would be the one. I have purposely memorized her number for this very reason. She is brilliant. Till this day, I don't know any other person who can completely learn a concept from sitting in just one class. Her intelligence and work ethic has led to her becoming a medical director before the age of thirty-five. She would never brag about that, but I never hesitate to shed light on her impressive accomplishments.

Kind

She calls me the hopeless romantic, but Ayo is the one with the heart of gold. Her kindness exudes in her relationships with friends and family. She always can see the good in people. She is my sounding board when I want to cut a tie. She will always give someone the benefit of the doubt. As I write this, I can hear her saying, "Well, Dee, did you consider . . . ?" She has taught me so much about selflessness. She does for others every single day and has never once complained about it. Living on her couch after one of my devastating breakups, I cried over burritos as Ayo listened emphatically. That generosity cannot be taught. It is in her DNA and is the reason she shines so brightly.

Fun

It is safe to say we share and embrace the motto, "Work hard, play hard!" Her humor and love of life is infectious. It permeates the room and instantly puts others at ease. Her honest take on life is so refreshing. Ayo is genuine. Most would think that she would have her nose in the air with so many successes under her belt. She never puts on airs or claims to be someone she's not. People love being around her energy . . . because it's real!

Almost twenty years later, she remains my confidante. Ayo is the person I can depend on for anything, be it career advice or just to chat about the ridiculous detox diet I just saw on TV. It was a touching moment to watch her walk down the aisle this past year. It was a feeling of happiness but also nostalgia to think of all the good guys, bad guys, awkward first dates, tears, and laughter of our dating history. We are now in our thirties and wives after fully enjoying (and learning) during our twenties. That decade was not only filled with building our medical knowledge but also with many years learning lessons about life, love, and what really matters.

Ayo will teach you about balance, which includes the importance of being a giver but not at the sacrifice of your own stability. She will discuss one of my favorite words: boundaries. You will see how you can shine as a role model but still possess the humility to keep your relationships sincere.

We are both psychiatrists. This means we have the privilege of seeing relationships from both our personal and professional perspectives. We have been the couples and family therapists. We can see what works in relationship dynamics and what doesn't. Thus, we soon realized that the questions we got most were about relationships, often from colleagues, friends, family, and patients. We decided to write this book to share our medical expertise with our personal relationship histories to provide solid advice for the wives reading and why our single ladies should not give up hope.

CHAPTER

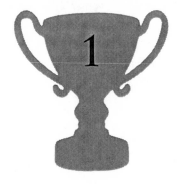

1

*"There is nothing
more appealing than a woman
who loves herself."*

THE MODERN TROPHY WIFE LOVES HERSELF

The traditional wife was once thought of as the woman who stayed at home and served her husband. She took care of the house and made sure he was comfortable when he got home from a long day's work. I remember the 1950s television sitcoms of mothers making sure all the family personal needs were met and the house was in tip-top shape. This was our society's model of a wife, one who was constantly giving. But when did this woman take care of herself? It is very easy to fall into the trap of just doing for others and neglecting ourselves.

As wives, mothers, and caretakers, we often put others' needs first. This is especially true of the resilient women who are taking care of parents in addition to their own families. It's a tough job with little recognition, and we must not neglect our own care to get it done. I've heard women say they feel guilty for taking time to just read a magazine at the end of the day. Are you kidding me? Ladies, taking time out for yourself is not selfish—it is necessary. The "all care, no play" formula does not work. It leads to women who are burned out, bored, and sometimes even resentful. One of the ways to show yourself some love is to take care of you, similar to how you show you love others by taking care of them.

1

Self-care is a key element in loving yourself, and it preserves your ability to function in and out of the home as a Modern Trophy Wife (MTW). You must learn how to love and focus on yourself, as we've been so engrained to do just the opposite.

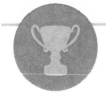

> **"Self-care is a key element in loving yourself, and it preserves your ability to function in and out of the home as a Modern Trophy Wife (MTW)."**

REFUEL YOUR OWN TANK

You cannot pour from an empty cup. Simplified, this means you can't give if you're not whole. How can you function when your tank is on empty? You need fuel! That fuel is self-care. I often hear that being a mother and/ or a wife can be a thankless job. Well, it's time to start applauding yourselves and regularly doing things to take care of *you*. One of the most important ways to thank yourself is to schedule time for refueling.

First, make a list of all the things you enjoy doing (outside of being with your spouse or kids). It can be anything. I'll share my list: going to the movies, pampering myself with manicures, waxes, and massages, and going out to dinner with my girlfriends. Next, figure out the frequency that you need to fill your tank. Here's my schedule:

- *Pamper:* one or two times a month
- *Dinner with girlfriends:* once every one or two months
- *Catch a movie:* once a week
  (yes, the movie theater is my local heaven)

After you have made your list, place it on your calendar or in your phone. I believe in the power of putting things in writing to make them a reality. Like I said, this is mandatory.

Now, your calendar is not to be filled with bad habits. I said self-care, not self-destruction. Binge-eating, heavy alcohol consumption, and pretty much anything that can result in you getting arrested are off the list. Those are extreme cases, but the same rule applies for pretty much anything that could result in stress. For example, I avoid gossiping and watching reality shows with fighting because it makes me feel heavy with bad emotions. I get tense and uneasy. If you get this same reaction with any particular activity, avoid, avoid, avoid.

Take a day off

We have all taken days off from work for doctor's appointments, to stay home with the kids, or to go to a family event. Guess what? Those don't count for your "me time." You may have used your paid time off for these things, but don't be fooled—those were working days. Here is my next request: I challenge you to take a day off from work to do what you want to do. It can be any day of the week. Send the kids to school and kiss your hubby goodbye. Then, it is "me time." You can do what makes you happy and feel at peace. It can be absolutely nothing. On some of my days off, I have stayed in my pajamas all day with the remote in one hand and popcorn in the other. It was heavenly. I also have spent days off catching a matinee, meeting a friend for lunch, or having a shopping excursion.

My only advice here is not to overschedule this day with too many activities. That becomes less soothing and more hectic. No matter what activity I choose, the important thing is that it makes me feel good. At the end of the day, I am happy and feel rested. It is often the refill that an MTW needs to return to being more productive at work and home.

Put the phone down

This might be the toughest challenge of all for my working ladies. However, if you do not need to have the phone on for anything work-related, I suggest trying a weekend day off from your conversations. This includes email, phone, *and* text. The beauty of technology is that people can reach you in a trillion ways ... direct message, email, Snapchat, Google Chat, phone chat, any type of chat. The downside is that it makes it harder to unplug from all of this. The days of just unplugging the house phone are prehistoric. However, you can put your phone down. I do this at times when I feel overwhelmed. It's perhaps my grown-up way of taking a time-out. Even though I didn't throw a tantrum to get there, I really do feel calmer when my time-out is over. As Modern Trophy Wives, we are playing the consistent juggling act between career and family. Every now and then, we need to step back and take a breather. Put the phone down, clear your mind, and do one of the self-care activities we've listed. You will return rejuvenated.

My advocation for self-care is not a plea to leave your families to fend for themselves. It is simply a reminder to take care of you. You absolutely must carve out time for yourself. Your body and mind will thrive and your family will appreciate the happier you.

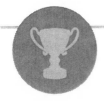 **" Make sleep a priority."**

MAKE SLEEP A PRIORITY: WIND DOWN BEFORE YOU FALL DOWN

Make sleep a priority. Did you know that when you're sleep deprived, you are more likely to eat unhealthy food, get irritable, and make mistakes? A good night's rest is needed not just for energy but also for memory and concentration. We are not college coeds anymore. The days of getting a couple hours of sleep and being able to fully function are long gone. We also no longer have the luxury of being able to take a three-hour nap in the afternoon. One of the best ways to ensure you prioritize your sleep is to wind down first.

A wind-down routine can never be overrated! Your wind-down routine is whatever you do one hour before bedtime. This is essential for a Modern Trophy Wife to reboot. Following a hard day's work, spending time with your hubby, or getting the kids to bed, all you want to do is just plop into the bed face first. Unfortunately, this does very little for overall relaxation and getting better-quality sleep.

Here are my tips to unwind:

1. **Avoid technology before bed.** Cell phones, television, and laptops can keep the brain wired when it's time to shut down.

2. **Do not take your work to bed.** You aren't going to be as productive, anyway. I wish I could get all those hours back that I tried to read textbook chapters in bed. I should have been sleeping so I could be alert and more productive for the next morning.

3. **Participate in a relaxing activity.** Take a warm bath, have a cup of soothing tea, or read a chapter from your favorite book in dim lighting in a nearby room—not in your bedroom. I encourage any activity that helps you decompress from the day.

4. **Bed is for sleep and sex only.** No exceptions.

This wind-down routine will provide you with a deeper sleep, which will promote better brain functioning the next day. Falling asleep will be easier, too. Making these changes is more effective in the long run than any sleeping pill, despite what their enticing commercials tell you. In fact, for a lot of people with sleep issues, implementing these changes can prevent the need for any prescription.

With that said, please sleep. Your body will thank you.

EXERCISE: MEDICINE FOR THE BODY AND MIND

There is no way you can read a book by two doctors without us tooting the horn about how awesome exercise is. You have heard the physical benefits of exercising for maintaining a healthy weight, lessening the risk of heart disease, and reducing the chances of developing chronic diseases. But there's more. Exercise is good for the body *and* the mind. The mood benefits are remarkable: exercise helps to lower anxiety, ease symptoms of depression, and boost energy. My patients would tell you that I'm like a broken record when I talk about the benefits of exercise. It works so well that I have to continually sing its praises. The reason behind its psychological effectiveness is related to endorphins. The brain releases endorphins during exercise, boosting our mood. For some women, exercise can have similar effects as antidepressant medications.

Motivation is the driving factor. I recognize that it is not easy for everyone to just jump up and start getting active. The hardest part is often getting started. With that said, here are some tips to help you get off the couch and get those sneakers on!

1. **Implement the buddy system**

   Exercising with others has helped me stay motivated. I am going to be honest: the gym and I were not on the best of terms a few years ago. I hated running and never picked up a weight. I would go to the gym only for aqua aerobics class, and ninety-five percent of the reason I went is because I wanted to be in the pool. This past year, I started trying new classes and meeting others with the same goals. I met other MTWs balancing career and family. On days I am reluctant or think about making something else a priority, these women keep me accountable.

2. **Find something you enjoy**

   Exercise just means that you're moving. You can walk, play tennis, do yoga, or dance. Don't like the gym? Walk around the mall, pop in a fitness DVD, or dust off the old exercise bike in the basement. There are so many options for ways to incorporate physical activity into your day. If you prefer sports, research leagues in your neighborhood. I got back into playing tennis at age thirty after a fifteen-plus-year hiatus. It has been one of the best decisions I have made for the decade. Pick something that you love and can stick to.

3. **Set realistic goals**

   Set a goal that you can accomplish. If you haven't worked out in more than a year, planning to go to the gym for five or six days a week right off the bat isn't going to work. You can start off by doing thirty minutes of activity two or three times a week and work from there. Remember, if your goals are too hard to attain, you are more likely to quit. Do not expect to lose twenty pounds in two weeks. And if you do, there is no way that's medically safe. It is best to set small, realistic goals to get more done in the long term. Slow and steady wins the race. Just keep moving!

THE POWER OF CONFIDENCE

A happier you is a more confident you. Confidence is sexy, magnetic, and immediately evident. You walk in the room and it grabs others' attention. Confidence is better than any crisp business card that you can hand out. It is a shining characteristic of a Modern Trophy Wife in the workplace and the home. Confidence is also the key to achieving more in your life. Those who have it are more likely to advance in their career. Does this mean they are smarter or more experienced? No! They just believe that they can do it.

Likewise, if you are insecure and always questioning your decisions, it is also apparent to those around you. This insecurity is contagious, and others will start to question your decisions. If you want to be a leader, you have to buck up. Ninety percent of being an effective leader is confidence. People trust leaders to make the big decisions because they believe they will get things done.

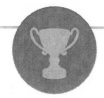

" People trust leaders to make the big decisions because they believe they will get things done."

Do you want to become a trailblazer in the workplace? That's simple. Bolster your self-esteem and be confident in your choices. If you have an idea to suggest at a meeting, speak up! When you arrive at a networking event, introduce yourself with a firm handshake; do not wait for someone to read your name tag to meet you. The confident person at the networking event is always the most memorable. Do you want to make vertical moves in the workplace but feel that you have been stagnant? Do a quick check of your workplace self-esteem meter:

Do you speak up at meetings or do you wait to be called on?

Do you propose new ideas?

Do coworkers come to you to make key decisions?

Do you introduce yourself at networking meetings?

When was the last time you got a promotion?

Have you ever discussed advancing with your employer?

If you haven't been pursuing any of the above, start by showing your confidence in just one of these areas at work this week. You want to be recognized as the go-to person. Displaying confidence will help you to not just keep your job but also to thrive at work. Thriving leads to more opened doors and a more fulfilling career. Start wearing that confidence!

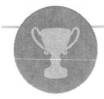

"A woman who knows what she wants and is not afraid to say it out loud is appealing."

In school, I hated public speaking. I dreaded those group projects where each student had to present in front of the whole classroom. This was a longtime fear, from my elementary school days up to my Power-Point presentations in medical school. I gave the same mediocre performance every time. My head was down, my were legs shaking behind the podium, and I would speed-read through the slides in 15 minutes to get it over. As I advanced in my career, I began teaching one-on-one not only my patients but also my family and friends, and I soon discovered that I really enjoyed it. It was incredibly gratifying for me to teach with the focus of helping others.

In time, I wanted to start doing it on a broader scale. I wanted to help more people through teaching, but I shuddered at the idea of public speaking. How was that going to work? I knew my past experience as a public speaker wouldn't fly. If I weren't a confident speaker, people would tune me out and not think that I had anything meaningful to say. I had to strengthen this weakness immediately to achieve my teaching dream.

I took control of the fear and joined Toastmasters, a group that promotes leadership and effective communication skills. On Saturday mornings, I stood in front of my Toastmasters group and spoke. As each meeting passed, my legs began to shake less, I began to slow down, and I even made eye contact with my audience. I gained more and more confidence in myself and what I had to say. People wanted to listen. At the end of the meetings, my audience wanted more. They wanted to know more about me and my expertise. Over time, I went from speaking to my Toastmasters group of twenty to speaking as an expert on live international television. This is the power of confidence. It is life changing, but I discovered this only because I recognized my weakness and faced it head-on.

What are you insecure about? What would help you become more confident in this area?

Confidence shines not only in the workplace but also at home. It is a key element for successful relationships. My husband once told me that confidence is the most attractive characteristic a woman can have. A woman who knows what she wants and is not afraid to say it out loud is appealing. Women who lack confidence often suffer with heightened anxiety, especially with making decisions. They are always fearful of what others may think and often depend on people to help them decide. They deal with feelings of self-blame and regret that can spiral into depression.

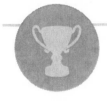

" Confidence is not just something to project for yourself but also for your marriage."

Confidence is not just something to project for yourself but also for your marriage. If you trust your husband and are assured that your union is stable, do not fall into the hole of suspicion. Do not let your past boyfriends' screwups affect your present relationship. If your husband has never given you a reason to think he has been unfaithful, why would you scroll through his call list? If he wants a guys' night, tell him to go for it. Your husband's healthy social life is just as important as your girls' night. He had friends before you tied the knot, and it is important to maintain those relationships while married.

Ladies, another important aspect of confidence in your marriage is maintaining your privacy. If you are confident in your marriage, then there is no reason to include others in your marital affairs. I have seen this go south very quickly where discussing the relationship with family and friends leads to gossip, hurt feelings, and, for some spouses, an abuse of trust. Have faith. If you know your marriage is strong, do not waste time looking for or causing cracks in the foundation. Hold your partner's hand

and proceed forth to conquer the world together. You are a great catch. Own it! Be confident in who you are, your marriage, your home, and your workplace. It's a winning formula.

" If you know your marriage is strong, do not waste time looking for or causing cracks in the foundation."

Confidence also sets a great example for your children. You are the first role models they have, so you must set a strong example. Kids watch and imitate us more than we realize. In my practice, I have seen children develop the same insecurities and social anxieties as their parents. There is a genetic component, but some of these are learned behaviors that the children have picked up from hearing their parents voice their fears. As Modern Trophy Wives pass on traits, why not let confidence be one of them? We all want confident children who can boldly reach for their dreams. This confidence starts within your home and the example you set.

Notes

CHAPTER

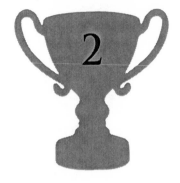

2

"Be intentional upon awakening from your dreams."

FROM THE DESK OF
Dr. Metzger

THE MODERN TROPHY WIFE HAS LIFE GOALS

Goals are a good thing. They inspire, guide, and, most important, they fulfill. Goals allow you to see your destination before you start your journey. Don't be timid when setting any life goals, whether in career, relationships, or health. The Modern Trophy Wife is a goal digger; not a gold digger. Stay true to your desires and set goals that *you* want to accomplish. There will be many twists and turns along the way, but your goals will be your compass leading you in the right direction. Have faith in your abilities and step forward. Achievement of set goals not only leads to feelings of happiness and accomplishment, but it also boosts confidence for further success.

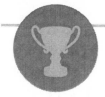

> **"The Modern Trophy Wife is a goal digger; not a gold digger."**

HEALTHIER HABITS

It is so easy for women to neglect their health when balancing responsibilities at home and work. A Modern Trophy Wife needs to be healthy to achieve all of this fabulousness. Eating unhealthy foods on-the-go and spending many hours sedentary at work doesn't do a body good.

13

The key to maintaining physical health is simply staying motivated. Humans are motivated by positive reinforcement. Children work to get a gold star on the bulletin board in school, and adults are not much different. In the world of fitness and diet, inches or pounds lost become our gold stars. Every time we see good results, that adds a little more to our motivation tank to keep going to the gym and avoiding eye contact with that frosted donut. We see the dream becoming a reality and we keep going.

So how do you stick to the goal of improved health? Make a schedule and stick to it—but make the schedule doable. Start off with what you can handle and build from there. You don't want to overwhelm yourself (physically or mentally) in starting a healthier diet and exercise plan; that's a sure recipe for early elimination. As you become more fit, you will realize that you are able to do more.

When you begin, set a goal and a timeline. The goal can be a certain weight, a clothing size, or even an activity. For instance, some of the goals I have set with patients include being able to walk a 5K, drink more water, or even smaller goals of being able to walk a flight of stairs without feeling winded. The importance is that the goal is something that makes you feel accomplished. Remember, diet and fitness goals are not just for you but also for your family. You want to be able to run outside with your grandchildren one day.

YOUR INNER CIRCLE

A healthy you is number one on your list of goals, and not far below are healthy relationships. When I turned thirty, I decided to make some goals for my relationships. I wanted to work on building the healthiest relationships I could. I also shifted my mentality from quantity to quality. I wanted to focus on spending time with those I held dear and detox from those I didn't. It was life changing. It made life much simpler and more positive. After marriage and kids, I began to value my time even more. Now, the central theme of prioritizing those I love and value is used to guide my relationship goals.

Another big relationship goal for me was to improve my communication. When I was younger, the principle of being right was most important. It didn't matter how much arguing it took, I always wanted to get my last word in. This would lead to heated debates and often end up with everyone involved feeling frustrated. In the aftermath, I would feel guilty about what I said and regret having the conflict in the first place. Therefore, I resteered my life to avoid recurring conflicts when possible. I now do best when I am quick to take responsibility for my actions and make apologies as needed. I no longer always have to be right.

The issue with always trying to be right is that it was closing my ears. I wasn't listening. So, I made it a goal to listen to those around me, to not interrupt and instead focus on what they were trying to express. I actually was able to pick up on more valid points with a resolution being much more possible. This goal has not only improved my relationship with my spouse, but also my relationships with family and friends. A huge amount of arguments are simply a result of miscommunication. A Modern Trophy Wife does better when she communicates better. It makes for a much more peaceful household.

These are just two of my goals, but there are many relationship goals you can add to the list. Goals can include having a biweekly date night with your husband, calling your college bestie at least once a month, or running far away from negative people. The company you keep has a huge influence on your mood and your success. As Dr. Gathing will later show you, your support system is a solid part of your foundation. Choose wisely.

THE MTW PROTOCOL: DREAM, BELIEVE, DO

Dream, believe, do has been my personal protocol since I finished medical school. It has worked for me and Dr. Gathing, along with our fellow Modern Trophy Wives. You cannot reach success without taking these three vital steps. You must dream it, believe you are capable, and then get it done.

Dream

"Dream big" is a popular slogan. The truth is that dreaming big is not enough—you have to *do*. Take some action. I love to use a kite analogy when I get into my dream talks with patients. An accomplished dream is equivalent to flying a kite. You have to put air under that kite to see it soar—and that air is action. What is the point of a kite that doesn't fly? It needs that gust of wind action to elevate it to new heights. In terms of your actions, I want you to put a whole wind machine under that thing. Dreams without any action are useless.

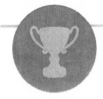

"The truth is that dreaming big is not enough—you have to *do*."

You first have to know what you're passionate about to figure out your dreams. I consider myself a dream catcher; I can't help it. If you tell me something you're passionate about, I will instantly want to hear your action plan. I always ask my patients about their interests and passions. I love to see their faces light up when they talk about them. But there are so many times when I ask, "What are your passions?" and hear the bewildered reply, "I don't know." If you are in that category, you have some pre-work to do.

In order to determine your passion, ask yourself these three things:

1. **What could you do every day that wouldn't feel like work? It can be anything.**
2. **As a child, what did you say you wanted to be when you grow up?**
3. **What do you like to do in your free time?**

Be careful to not confuse your gifts and your passions. They sometimes do not align. Being good at something doesn't necessarily mean you are passionate about it. You can be a gifted piano player who can play music by ear, but if you find playing to be a chore and have no interest in even owning a piano, it is not a passion. A passion is something that gives you pure joy. It never feels like a task, and you are always looking forward to the next opportunity to do it. You must be careful not to pursue something for reasons other than your own joy. Those reasons can include trying to please others, wanting money, or being good at something. The issue with any of those is that the drive eventually disappears if you lack the passion. That wind machine under the kite soon turns into a handheld fan until eventually the kite takes a nosedive.

Once you have identified your passion, the next step is to believe. Believing is what propels you to action.

Believe

We live in a world of excuses. I have started to despise the word *but* because it is almost always followed by an excuse. I'll hear "Doc, I would love to pursue that *but*..." It puts the emergency brake on dreams and brings them to a painfully screeching halt. It is time to kick the *buts* to the curb. Excuses are plentiful yet they serve no positive purpose in the life of a Modern Trophy Wife. They only slow down your progress. Please believe me—several *buts* come to mind at 5 a.m. when I don't feel like getting out of bed to exercise. However, my belief overrides those excuses. That belief that I can be fit and healthy gets my sneakers on and my behind in the car before the sun rises. You have to believe and shut those excuses down.

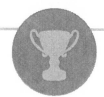

"**Excuses are plentiful yet they serve no positive purpose in the life of a Modern Trophy Wife.**"

Here are the most common excuses I hear. They make up what I call the Common Offenders List. As you can see, they usually start with "I don't have..." or "I'm too..."

"I don't have time." You have a husband who travels, a full-time job, and/or a full house of kiddies. It seems like the extra hours are diminishing by the second. Listen, a Modern Trophy Wife was not made to live life just to work and pay bills. Neither are our lives meant to be mediocre or convenient. We are given passions to

explore them. There is nothing sadder than an unpursued dream. Go for it, and *find* time to pursue those dreams. We can always find time for things we love. That's why I always followed that rule that if a man wasn't calling me, he wasn't interested. It's simple as that. If you truly love it, you will find time to pursue it.

"I don't have the money." This is a huge one. I have tried to use this excuse myself to block me from pursuing my dreams. My advice, which is also my personal testimony, is to just *start*. You have to start somewhere in your pursuit. I am a strong believer that when you pursue what is in your heart, the money will come. In the meantime, take it one day at a time. Take it one dollar at a time. If you think too far ahead about what you can and cannot afford, anxiety will consume you. Just focus on today, and you will notice an interesting phenomenon: doors will start opening as the days go on. In the words of Dory of *Finding Nemo*, you have to "just keep swimming." Invest what you've got and put your all in, and things will start happening. No risk, no reward!

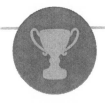

"There is nothing sadder than an unpursued dream."

"I'm too old." This should be officially banned as an excuse. You are never too old to find joy. In my opinion, the older you are, the faster you need to find it. If you are physically and mentally able to pursue a dream, you are not too old. Do you have a passion to be an artist? If so, can you lift a paintbrush? Then you're not too old. We cannot relive our glory days, but we can claim the bliss of today. Life is short, so let's make the most of our stay here. Forget your age and do what you love. What do you have to lose?

"I have tried and failed." Failure is a prerequisite to success. It's just part of the game. I have had more failures than I can count on two hands. The reality is that I don't view them as failures. I see

them as lessons and detours that steered me in the right direction. For all those frivolous failures, the successes have been big . . . actually, huge. In the end, I have realized that those closed doors were all part of the divine plan. I walked away from every closed door with more knowledge than I had before. This knowledge all contributed to my success. Bottom line: if you tried and failed, try again. Your history of failures will make the success that much sweeter. It will also provide a great inspiration to others who follow in your path.

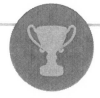

"Failure is a prerequisite to success."

"Everyone will think I'm nuts for doing this." This is an actual quote that I have heard too many times. You know what's really nuts? Somebody having the power over your life decisions. Passion is personal. No one can tell you where your joy is, nor can they give you directions to find it. If you love it, go for it. You have to let go of seeking others' approval. I say passion is personal because very often, other people can't see the spark that you do in the dream. You are looking through two very different lenses hoping for the same view, but that's impossible. Life does not work that way. If anyone has something negative to say about your dreams, tell them to take a hike. You don't need them blocking the wind for your kite, anyway.

Excuses aside, the moral of the story is that you have to believe it can happen. A Modern Trophy Wife is confident and talented. You must envision yourself engulfed in the world of your passion. See the kite soaring up in the sky. It looks nice, right? Envision your dream this way every single day.

Do

You know your passion...check. You believe it can be done...check. The next step is to make a deposit into that dream to start working toward your goal. Have a plan.

First, make a list and write it down. I can't emphasize enough the importance of putting your goals to paper. It makes them more concrete and attainable. Write it in your planner, in a journal, in your phone, on a sticky note, in lipstick on your mirror—it doesn't matter where as long as it is written somewhere you can see it. For example, let's say your passion is interior design. You have designed your own home beautifully and realized that you loved everything about the process. You have always been more drawn to the showcased interiors of HGTV than prime-time television. You have found the passion, so now it's time to pursue it. Here is my action plan proposal for this example:

1. **Look up local interior designers online and make contact.** One amazing thing that I have discovered in the world of medicine as well as media is that it never hurts to reach out. You never know who will reply and become a resource, an inspiration, or even a mentor. There are people in the world who like to pay it forward. These shining stars enjoy sharing their knowledge and being a blessing to others. You may just link with one of these stars. Now, be prepared for some radio silence when you send out those emails. That is just part of the process. Some will not respond, but remember that all it takes is one solid reply to get you to the next step.

2. **Research different styles of design.** Which appeals to you the most? Do you prefer modern or traditional? In order to sell yourself, you have to know who you are. What would be on your business card? Would you like to design homes, offices, hotels, or all of the above? If you have a niche, this is the time to claim it. It will assist you in finding others with the same interests.

3. **Get your interior design license and start taking pictures of your work.** If you want to go for it, you have to show off your skills!

I have said this before: confidence is more than half the battle. Believe that you're good, and the customers will come. People want an interior designer who knows her stuff and has a specific style. Display that in your pictures and also in how you present yourself. Act like you are the real deal.

If you follow this protocol of dream, believe, and do, your dreams will start becoming real. Opportunities will come from places you least expect. One thing that has amazed me is how one phone call or connection can catapult you further. One phone call with a producer propelled me from hosting a local television show in Atlanta to sitting on a panel of experts for a worldwide network. Don't underestimate how far these steps can take you. You will take small baby steps along the way, but you also will take huge leaps on the road to your destiny. Keeping faith is a key factor to staying on this road.

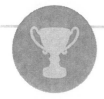

" Sometimes things will look dark, and you will want to throw in the towel. Faith, however, will be your lantern."

There will be times in your life when things are going to defy logic or explanation. They will bring you steps forward or backward. Have faith that the universe will bring you to your destiny. Have you ever felt disappointment when you didn't get a promotion, didn't get to move to a city you wanted to move to, or after a relationship abruptly ended? I'm sure you can remember the devastation you felt at the time. Now fast-forward to the present—do you still feel devastated? Can you see that maybe these doors were closing because better doors were opening down the hallway? Can you see this was part of a bigger plan? The belief that things are working for your good despite bad things happening is the definition of faith. It is the belief that you will still meet your life goals despite not being sure of exactly how you will do it.

Faith is essential for a Modern Trophy Wife. Sometimes things will look dark, and you will want to throw in the towel. Faith, however, will be your lantern.

A takeaway point about getting things done is that distractions and goals don't mix. You must always stay in grind mode as if your breakthrough may happen tomorrow. This will keep you on task. Having self-discipline is what separates the good from the great. This is my recipe for success. **Set life goals, work hard, stay faithful, achieve them, and repeat.** Goals written down and set with a timeline will help keep you accountable.

People often ask me how I got to the milestones in my career while balancing motherhood and marriage. I have no superhuman powers, nor do I have more time than others (I believe in getting seven to eight hours of sleep nightly). I simply followed the Modern Trophy Wife Protocol: **dream, believe, and do.** This is what will keep *your* kite soaring among the clouds, too.

Notes

CHAPTER

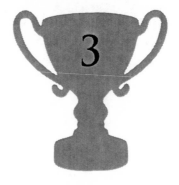

3

"The true meaning of life is finding the balance in who you are and what you do."

THE MODERN TROPHY WIFE BALANCES ROLES

I enjoy talking with women, being in their presence. I admire their beauty, their versatility, their strength. Whether personally or professionally, discussing women's unique life experiences and core beliefs interests me. And even more fascinating than our differences are the similarities I've observed.

One area that women in all walks of life seem to contend with is the concept of balance. In talking with friends or meeting with patients, I've heard statements such as, "I just have too much on my plate" or "I just can't be everything to everybody." Women often feel pressured to assume multiple roles, and they struggle to live up to a variety of expectations. Whether a girlfriend or wife, employee or manager, daughter or mother, you are regularly confronted with scenarios that present competing priorities. Your husband has a romantic weekend planned, but your aging parents need a caretaker. Your boss asks you to work late just as you were leaving to pick the kids up from day care. Or you finally planned a girls' night out but your little one starts running a fever.

Does any of this sound familiar? Are you constantly frustrated and overwhelmed with your day-to-day obligations? Do you feel like you are always letting someone down? Ladies, it is time to ditch the guilt!

As a Modern Trophy Wife, you are constantly seeking to improve your life as well as the lives of those around you. You have numerous obligations and strive to fulfill extraordinary expectations. This sense of ambition, of purpose, can lead to emotional and physical strain if not directed appropriately. As Dion mentioned, it is essential for you to take care of yourself before caring for others. But your nurturing nature is often focused on everyone but yourself.

Many of you have asked for guidance on how to manage all of the responsibilities you have taken on. Through my research and experience, I have deciphered the key factors involved in achieving balance when juggling various roles that we as Modern Trophy Wives assume. Ladies, it can be done. In this chapter, I will tell you how to create some stability in a world full of chaos.

BE IN THE MOMENT

Last year, I attended a seminar based on change model principles. The senior leadership at my job thought it would be good for us to participate in a session where we identified the hindrances in our current processes, and we explored the acceptance of the status quo. The idea was that once we were aware of what limited us, our motivation to change our outlook and actions would increase. As a behavioral health professional, I was fully open to the experience. Most topics seemed irrelevant, but I hung in there. Just when I thought that it could all go in one ear and out the other, a statement struck a chord with me: "Be here now."

I paused and took a minute to reflect on the idea. The session trainers proposed that what makes an interaction meaningful is that you are present in that moment, giving the situation or individual your full attention. This concept was contrary to my usual strategy for complicated situations and a hectic schedule—multitasking. Like most women, I believe that multitasking is a strength. I can run a Web meeting, write an email, and plan my next workout without missing a beat. I was convinced that I gave the perfect amount of attention to everything I worked on. It seemed very effective for me, especially in the workplace. Or so I thought.

The trainer presented evidence that when you think you're giving a task or interaction enough attention, you likely aren't.

When I arrived home that night, I told my husband about what I learned. I mentioned the ridiculous directive we were given to focus on just one thing at a time in all areas of life for the next few weeks. If sending an email, complete that email. If on a conference call, concentrate on that call. And so forth. I told him that I was the queen of multitasking and felt they were misguided in trying to alter this routine. He laughed at that. When I gave him a confused expression, he explained, "Babe, you constantly miss things. You don't always listen." I was shocked. Appalled even. The nerve of him to accuse me of not being a good listener!

But after hearing him out, I reviewed his scenarios. Eating dinner while scrolling through my calendar; checking my email while cuddled up watching movies; and maybe worst of all, the conference calls while at the gym. Maybe he had a point. Maybe there was a piece of these moments I was missing with my mind being elsewhere. Or more likely, there were some things others weren't getting while I was multitasking.

So I decided to give focused attention a try. I couldn't abandon multitasking altogether, but if there were moments that I needed to be engaged or in tune with those around me, I attempted to be in that moment. When my coworkers came into my office, I stopped what I was doing and listened. When my husband told a story about his unreliable employees, I listened to the details and gave constructive feedback. When my team presented in a Web meeting, I stopped working on other projects to focus on the task at hand. The results were incredible! Not only did I retain more information from my encounters, but the people in my life could tell that I was more engaged. They casually mentioned how amazed they were that I was putting my phone down for more than a second, or that I didn't say "huh?" at all during a conversation.

My mini experiment was complete and the results were in. Not only did I get just as much done during this time, but I also felt more confident as I knew exactly what was put into the task at hand. This was not rocket science, but it definitely changed the game for me.

You are a motivated woman, so there is always a lot to do and squeeze in. Naturally, you use multitasking as a coping strategy. You have a strict deadline due, but your toddler wants to be rocked to sleep "only by

Mommy." You need to meal-prep to avoid your second food truck trip this week, but your bestie wants to rehash every detail of her latest date. So what is a girl to do? Before, I would've said throw that baby on one knee with that computer on the other; or hold that phone on your shoulder and get to meal-prepping! But not now. One of the best approaches to building and strengthening relationships is to pay attention and spend quality time. This applies not just to your personal life but also professionally.

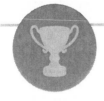

> " One of the best approaches to building and strengthening relationships is to pay attention and spend quality time."

Quality time doesn't have to be lengthy or in a particular setting. It is simply an interaction with limited interruptions. It is great when these exchanges fit within your schedule or never-ending to-do list, but they are often unscripted. You have to be aware of what someone needs from you in those moments and prioritize him or her. Using these interfaces to attend to others can take you further than a handful of preoccupied exchanges.

Ladies, I know what you're thinking. With all the responsibilities you have and expectations to live up to, giving up multitasking would be absurd. And if you are anything like me, your brain is constantly racing with thoughts, and it is hard to shut them off. I have about 100 notes in my phone with all sorts of tidbits and to-do lists. However, taking an active interest in whoever is in front of you, even if for a short period, can show that you care and that they are worthy of your time. Is a ten-minute delay in responding to that email really going to be detrimental? Is running that Google image search on the perfect outfit for your big presentation in the morning really more important than reading to your child? And don't get me started on how scrolling through Facebook can ruin any intimate moment with just one hilarious video!

Convenience and immediate gratification have become the norm. It's now perfectly acceptable to spend "quality time" with your coworkers or loved ones while multitasking, especially with technology and social media involved. But what we are really doing is giving a bit of ourselves to pacify each situation instead of giving someone or some task the attention deserved.

As a Modern Trophy Wife, it is important to prioritize important interactions. Be present with those attempting to communicate with you. Truly engage. Turn off the autopilot. Stop sending back text replies in the middle of a conversation, or watching television during family dinnertime. These are the moments of opportunity that you can make someone feel loved or special; they can go a long way in making yourself and those around you feel more satisfied in the relationship.

Give it a try. Start out with just one week of devoting your full attention to the tasks and persons that you encounter. Go ahead. *Be there.*

WIFEY VS. MOMMY

The most challenging roles to balance for a Modern Trophy Wife are those of wife and mother. It all starts with being so in love with someone that you can't imagine life without him. You can't stop thinking about him. You anticipate every encounter. You hurt when he hurts. You decide that he is the one for you and there is no one else in the world you would rather go through the ups and downs of life with. Like you, he feels the two of you are written in the stars, and you resolve to become husband and wife. You work out the kinks and accept each other's flaws; communication finally becomes second nature. That's when it happens. You agree that it is time to expand your family. And that is where things start to get complicated.

Being a nurturer, supporter, and confidante to your spouse while raising your child or children can be extraordinarily difficult. Your infant is born as an innocent being and representation of the love you have for one another, so it is easy to place your entire focus on your child. And who would blame you? Infants are completely dependent and unable to care for themselves. They rely on you for protection and survival. And of course fathers have a major place in childrearing, but there is nothing like the bond between mother and newborn. You just melt when you look into that little face or smell that sweet baby smell. And on the worst day when the crying is nonstop, the poop keeps coming, and you can't remember the last time you've showered, you still have a little energy left to stare at your little one sleeping.

So there you are, reading your parent guides, trying to maintain your emotions and not lose your sleep-deprived mind, when your husband reminds you that he exists. You try to grasp a recollection of the time when you were head over heels, when there was nothing more important in the entire world than being with him, but the memories elude you. And if you can remember those moments and play them back, the feelings that used to correspond have somehow changed. You look into his eyes and see the man who used to be your everything, but instead of daydreaming about going in for a kiss, you just pray he will relieve you for a nap.

Best-case scenario, your man is as patient as he can be. Telling you how beautiful you look while your hair mattes up. Cooking whatever he knows how to so you can have a break. But the time will come when he looks to you with that longing eye. He wants it back; he wants *you* back. He wants his sex kitten, his partner in crime, and the love of his life to be the person he fell in love with. He wants to start facing the world together again; he wants you to have his back. And you want to be that girl who loved so freely and completely when you made your relationship a priority. But your little perfect angel *needs* you, not just *wants* you.

"You can be an amazing wife, devoted mother, and maintain your sanity."

Ladies, you are not alone. Trying to take care of yourself while balancing wifehood and motherhood can feel like an impossible juggling act. You end up neglecting your own needs in an effort to feel successful in your other roles, which further exacerbates the situation as you have less motivation and energy to attend to your loved ones. Do not despair. You can be an amazing wife, devoted mother, and maintain your sanity. You are a Modern Trophy Wife, and that means you can do this, and do it with grace. And I am going to help you!

BALANCING TIPS FOR WIFEY AND MOMMY

1. Maintain a sense of self

You may not remember what your life was like before you got married or had children. You get flashbacks or déjà vu, but it seems like lifetimes ago that you were able to think about only you or focus on your sole desires. And when was the last time you were alone, truly alone, with enough silence to hear a pin drop? In a life filled with piano lessons and dinner parties, you often forget to put yourself on the agenda. When was the last time you were able to concentrate on your own feelings and listen to your own thoughts? Over time, this starts to cause a lack of self-awareness. Life keeps moving and changing, so you need to remain in tune with your own voice to ensure you are comfortable with the person you see when you look in the mirror.

At least once per month, arrange a time for inner reflection. Where you can be self-focused. Away from the hubby, kids, and responsibilities. Away from your friends, siblings, and coworkers. You have learned that these private moments are reserved for refueling your empty tank and pouring into yourself. But that is not all. In these moments, you can confirm you are living your truth and fulfilling your own purpose. You can do this in many ways, including prayer, meditation, or writing down creative ideas and goals. As you see, I did not mention television, social media, or movies. These do not promote introspection. Activities that allow you to get caught up in the lives or stories of others do not allow you to be one with your own thoughts. Find an outlet that centers you and gets you to a place where you feel like your best self. Make time to do that thing—yourself!

You may never have been a person who likes to be alone. You thrive on being around others. For you, being alone leads to boredom or feeling like you are missing something. You dread the idea of time to yourself. This may be a sign of a larger issue. People who do not like to be alone are more likely to struggle with insecurity or poor self-esteem, and less able to cope with negative emotions. We all experience loneliness at times as humans innately seek companionship, but the inability to self-soothe or manage negative feelings may be a symptom of trauma, grief, depression, or anxiety. Those who live a healthy, balanced life are able to work through downfalls or emotional setbacks and move forward using their resources. Seek help in a trusted friend, counselor, or spiritual mentor if you need assistance in working through these difficulties.

2. Do not neglect wifey duties

Marriage is about two people giving 100 percent of their energy toward being together. This does not change when someone gets a new job, when time has passed, or when children come. I often wondered why marriage was called an institution, but I now know why. An institution is an establishment, an organization that needs as much cultivation as any business or enterprise. So why then do we feel lackadaisical or even ashamed of making our marriage a priority? If I tell my friends that I can't go hang out because I have to work late, there are no questions asked. But let me say it's because I need to spend quality time with my husband and I get frowns or blank stares. When Chrissy Teigen went out with her husband during her newborn's second week of life, she was slandered. Since when did careers and children take precedence over something that we swore to protect at all costs?

Society has begun to deem marriage "a dying institution." Men and women alike have started to speak negatively about the custom, calling it old-fashioned and outdated. But I contend that two people spending their lives together, taking on whatever life hands them, is no more outdated than the concept of making money doing what you love. I think people have grown reluctant to put time and energy into something that is not a sure thing, in something they cannot control. We live in a time where people want certainty and immediate gratification for the work they do, not to have faith and be loyal through ups and downs. And by "they" I mean *you*. You want to be in, but not all in. You want a marriage, but not the years of effort. You want a husband, but don't want to be sensitive to his needs.

I have worked with many wives who have put more energy into planning their wedding than they did in their first year of marriage. This is preposterous. It is time to get back to basics. It's time to get back to seeing marriage as an entity that needs constant attention and nurturing. This may be a traditional way of thinking, but there is no other way for two people to last in a marriage other than being fully dedicated. I am not saying to neglect your livelihood or children, but just recognize that you have a duty as a wife just like you do as an employee or a mother. It can't take a backseat to anything else in your life. And this is not important for just you and your husband. Your children need to see their parents communicating and working together as a team. They need to see what love and commitment look like. You are a model of how they should act and be treated within relationships.

So what are these duties, you ask? Here is the "wifey" job description:

- *Be your husband's biggest fan.* Men do not receive much positive reinforcement in life, so a man's wife is the one person he can count on to encourage and praise him. You have to be his ultimate champion and cheerleader. When I tell wives this in couple's therapy, they frequently ask, "Why a cheerleader? Why can't I be his teammate?" Men already have teammates in life—in their jobs, sports, or creative projects. But it is rare that a man has a cheerleader. Someone rooting for him against all odds and believing in him even when things don't look possible. You have to be that for your husband. The person who lets him know that win or lose, you will be there, continuing to motivate him even when you are upset or frustrated.

  As a Modern Trophy Wife, this can be a challenge. You are used to being the one who receives praise and adoration, not giving it. You do not know how to put your ego aside and be the supporter your husband needs. Your first assignment is to learn how. You can start by remembering how you did that when you were dating.

- *Maintain an intimate relationship with your husband.* Yes, this includes sex, but that is not all. Intimacy is closeness, a friendship that develops over time. It encompasses the mental, physical, and emotional aspects of a relationship and requires continual nurturing. To remain intimate with your husband requires spending quality time away from friends, family, and children in an effort to foster the relationship. Intimacy means doing things together that you enjoy, praying together, and remembering why you fell for each other in the first place. Limiting the focus on the children or work and talking about common interests and future life goals builds attachment and provides a "check-in" on the relationship. These loving moments encourage vulnerability in your emotions and reinforce a connection that no one else shares.

" Maintaining sex appeal and compatibility is just as much about confidence as it is about physical attraction."

And of course, maintaining a fun and open sexual relationship is essential. You have to be willing to experiment and be unguarded with your husband. After all, the two became one flesh, so your body is his body! Maintaining sex appeal and compatibility is just as much about confidence as it is about physical attraction. Try not to fixate on your looks or weight; own your body and be comfortable in your own skin. If there is work you want to do to become healthy, definitely take action, but while you do the work just know that your confidence and attentiveness to his physical needs will prevail.

• *Continue to anticipate your husband's needs.* It sounds simple and probably used to be in the beginning, but it has likely fallen off a bit over time, especially after becoming a mommy. In fact, this skill of anticipating needs has been sharpened and honed in motherhood. You know when your child will be hungry so you pack an extra snack. You know to put that Pull-Up on for long car rides and that special blanket in the bag to avoid World War III. So why do we start to lose these senses when it comes to our husband? You used to make his favorite dinner when he was having a bad day, tape the game for him when his meetings ran long, or wear his favorite nightie on date night. Now you can't remember the last time you made more than a three-ingredient meal or even wore a thong. Being thoughtful and considerate will go a long way in showing your husband that he is important and a priority.

3. **Silence your biggest critic**

One of the conditions of perfection is that there is no room for improvement. That there are no flaws or faults. To be human, however, means that you will make mistakes and have errors in judgment. So it is important to remember that when you approach any role in life. As a wife and mother, you will make numerous mistakes and feel like a failure. But you are not alone! There is no perfect way for two people to come together and build a life together, and there is definitely no perfect way to parent a child. As a Modern Trophy Wife, you are constantly seeking to enrich yourself and the world, but you cannot confuse striving for improvement with striving for perfection.

"You cannot confuse striving for improvement with striving for perfection."

Often, the need to strive for perfection comes from feeling imperfect. This can stem from a deep-rooted and subconscious fear that you are not good enough, or perhaps because you feel inferior to others. The attempt to be perfect is a response to these internal fears and often a reflection of the insecurities. Believing that you can achieve perfection leads to failure, and that reinforces negative thoughts. This can become a pattern and, if not evaluated, even an obsession. Some feelings of inferiority in various circumstances can be normal and can motivate you to grow and do better. But when perfectionism becomes a fixation and limits your ability to be content with yourself and your life, it can lead to anxiety, depression, or self-destructive behavior.

To prevent the vicious cycle of perfectionism and self-defeating thoughts, you have to develop a sense of self-worth. Once you realize the amazing person that you are and know that you are good enough, you will begin to tolerate simple mistakes. You will be able to tolerate the idea that you have flaws. You can then finally silence your biggest critic, your own inner voice.

Recognizing your strengths as well as your weaknesses is the first step to self-improvement and the key to moving forward. If you are looking at your current situation as a disappointment, then you likely are not able to feel pleased in the day-to-day moments with your loved ones. In striving for perfection, you are not allowing yourself to enjoy the present. Identifying areas for improvement yet being assured in your journey provides the balance you need to bring contentment to your life.

4. Make mommy playdates

Playdates. They were developed for children to strengthen their social skills and avoid isolation while spending their primary time within their family system. The days of children in the community coming together on a regular basis with kids in the neighborhood have been replaced with video games and tablets. You may be experiencing a similar phenomenon in your life. Keeping up with your day-to-day is causing a lack of social interaction and isolation. Your usual outlet—getting together regularly with your friends and loved ones outside of your nuclear family—has been replaced by social media and electronic devices. You are likely stuck in the rigmarole of your daily life.

It is time for mommy playdates. And I do not mean coming together and exchanging pleasantries with the moms of your children's friends while they hang out. No! I am talking about reaching out to your friends and loved ones, your trusted companions, and arranging an outing. Friends coming together as friends to provide entertainment and reassurance for one another. After the kiddie talk and obligatory photo sharing, you can start with play. This is when you get to let your hair down, de-stress, and enjoy yourself. Swap stories, provide encouragement, and give feedback. Talk about things you could never discuss in front of your children, or that your husband would never be interested in. You may just learn some new recipes, secrets, or tricks. And if you are lucky, you will have a ton of laughs. There is nothing more crucial than sharing your thoughts with like-minded individuals and knowing that you have support. That you are not alone.

Having this time away from your daily routine and from your family allows you to take some space and appreciate them. You can then go back with a sense of renewal.

So stop putting it off and plan that mommy playdate!

5. Develop your individualized life plan

As discussed earlier, one of the most important aspects of being a Modern Trophy Wife is developing your life goals. But this is an area that may need to be reinvented. Before you got married or had children, you had a dream. You had an idea of what your life would be like. You may have achieved those dreams prior to getting married and having children, and you must now accommodate your new roles into your former vision. Or maybe you derailed your dreams to focus on your family life and need to redefine your purpose. Now is the time to start dreaming again. Reclaim your life. Are you on track with where you want to be physically? Do you need to obtain further experience or training to get back into the workforce? What do you want your marriage to be like?

There are so many areas that you need to analyze in order to develop your life plan, but the main concept is to not lose sight of your own dreams. You do not want to wake up one day and realize that you put all of your eggs in one basket when you had other aspirations. To get back on track, you need to visualize where you want to be and design a plan to get there. This plan may include ideas for your personal, professional, social, and emotional well-being. Many of these areas may coincide. Getting your sexy back and joining a running group may reinforce your personal and social goals. Going to a couple's therapist to reconnect with your husband could improve your personal life and emotional well-being. Or changing your career and following through with your passion project may revitalize your professional life and stabilize your finances. And so on and so forth.

Whether it is plans for tomorrow or for the next five years . . . Dream. Believe. Do.

Notes

CHAPTER

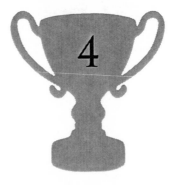

4

*"Pursue your destiny
by making your own rules."*

THE MODERN TROPHY WIFE MAKES HER OWN RULES

Women have more choices than ever regarding what to do with our lives. We can pursue higher education, patron the arts, or create tech start-ups. We can be young parents, delay motherhood, or choose to be childless. Because we can earn a living wage in various industries, we are no longer confined to a limited set of choices. Modern Trophy Wives are embracing our personal and professional freedoms, exploring options that were restricted in the past. Female integration into all levels of the workforce has been exciting and empowering, yet it creates new interpersonal challenges. Broadening the opportunities that lie before us hasn't changed our fundamental drive to nurture. It hasn't silenced some of our biological clocks. And it definitely hasn't changed the inflexible culture of some workplaces.

This can create a conflict in how we choose to define ourselves, in whom we choose to become. We may start to second-guess ourselves and lack confidence in our ability to achieve certain goals. This insecurity is constantly reinforced by society and those around us. We begin to live by a certain set of guiding principles that we didn't define for ourselves. Subliminal messages shape our belief that we need to strive for a certain physical ideal, that we can't thrive in certain settings, or that we must choose between a successful career and a family. Don't even get me started on the newest craze to freeze eggs earlier and earlier "just in case." Just in case what? In case our knight in shining armor never shows up?

I can't count how many pitiful looks I received when discussing relationships before I got married or how many times I've heard, "You don't have a baby yet? What are you waiting for?" It was mostly from other women! For so long we were put into a box with our paths predetermined that it is difficult for some to see that there may be other viable options. Our culture has not fully evolved to incorporate the innumerable possibilities that we may develop as our sense of purpose.

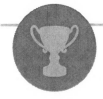

" Ladies, you have to resist the labels and false messages that others attempt to impose."

Ladies, you have to resist the labels and false messages that others attempt to impose. You have to define who you want to be personally and professionally. You must define your own rules and live by them. This means listening to your own voice and discovering your own ideals, which may differ from those of your family, friends, and society. You can't establish your own values and ambitions while looking at someone else's life, and definitely not by their social media page. Self-discovery involves looking within and determining how you perceive the world. You decide your beliefs on important topics such as spirituality, love, marriage, motherhood, politics, friendship, careers, and more. No more aligning with the expectations or pressures of others.

Here is a guide to get you started on your journey to self-discovery and some tips for creating your own rules!

SELF-AWARENESS

The first step in defining your own rules and taking control of your life is to become more self-aware. Self-awareness is the ability to be conscious of your own thoughts, feelings, and character. This means you know the basic answer to the question, "Who am I?" It seems like a simple concept;

however, we often focus on what is going on outside of us and not inside. We regularly examine what we are experiencing, but not what we think or feel. It is rare that we examine our beliefs and intentions consistently and often.

You constantly have a million thoughts in your head and a million and one things to do. You don't always have the time or energy to be introspective. You may catch yourself just going, doing, and reacting. And this is on a normal day. At other times, you are overwhelmed by the people and random tasks that need your attention. But to know who you are and to develop who you want to be, you have to be more focused on inner experiences. Being curious about what you believe and questioning the motivation behind your actions is the key to self-examination and growth. Do you find that the decisions you make are based on what you have always done or what your parents taught you? Or, more commonly, are they based on what others think? These are signs of limited self-awareness and that you are not living by your own rules. But that can change today.

A Modern Trophy Wife looks at every experience as one to learn about herself. Everyday situations can be used to provoke self-reflection and trigger opportunities for growth. In particular, you may uncover irrational thoughts that affect your behavior and guide your expectations of others. These wrong perceptions, known as cognitive distortions, can be self-defeating and damaging if not recognized. Cognitive distortions are especially important in intimate relationships, but they are relevant in all interactions. For example, you might think a man should always pay for everything and be the primary provider for the household. Or you think your boss should give praise regularly but minimize constructive negative feedback. Have you ever stopped to think about where these beliefs come from?

It is common for people to develop judgments based on past experiences and leave their distorted thoughts unchecked. This leads to unhealthy behavior patterns that affect your relationships with others. In the examples previously mentioned: If you make double the salary of your partner, is it not appropriate for you to make major purchases and be the breadwinner of the family? Or if your boss never addresses your weaknesses, how will you focus your development?

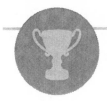

"A Modern Trophy Wife looks at every experience as one to learn about herself."

Once you become more mindful of your mindset and how you relate to others, you can start the process of self-correction. A simple way to start the process of self-correction is to challenge the thoughts you identify as leading to negative feelings and behaviors. Look at your beliefs from an objective perspective by examining the evidence as to why it may or may not be an effective thought process. You will begin to gain clarity regarding the viewpoints that have been causing stress or holding you back. Now you will be in a better position to identify the adjustments you need to make in order to take control of your life. This will in turn improve your cognizance in relationships. You will learn to break the patterns of negative thoughts that lead to negative behaviors, and you will finally start seeing more positive results.

IDENTIFY WHAT FULFILLS YOU

I knew I wanted to be doctor from the moment I could play with a stethoscope. My mother always says that it was amazing how early I expressed that desire and never wavered from it. I thought I wanted to specialize in pediatrics for a long time, but hey, I wasn't too far off! This sort of early clarity in a chosen career path is very rare. You may likely still be examining whether the direction you took is right for you, or maybe you are still trying to understand your calling. A career can be like a pair of designer heels. It looks great on the outside, like it was made for you. It seems to go well at first. Then you get into it for a while, and everything about it feels wrong. Like those too-high designer pumps, the career becomes uncomfortable and unsettling, and you just want to get out of it as quickly as possible. But you are worried about what people would think or how it would look. You worry that things may get worse if you make a change. So you keep it going and bear the pain, all the while knowing it isn't right for you.

If you are ready to try a new career, please know that it is a completely ordinary feeling! As Dion mentioned earlier, finding your passion is often a process. What works for someone else may not work for you. Sometimes you just have to "try on" different areas like you do shoes, looking for the right fit.

Unfortunately, once you discover what works for you, there may be other obstacles. You are still left to determine who you want to *be* apart from what you *do*. Practicing medicine has been a dream come true for me, but that does not complete my story. Upon reaching my life goal, I soon felt that there was more to accomplish, more living for me to do. However, at that point, unlike Dion, I had no blueprint, no roadmap. This created a conundrum, as my life decisions had always been completely directed toward becoming a doctor. After attaining that goal, for the first time in my life I had no apparent purpose. Was being the best psychiatrist I could be going to be enough? Was there something more out there for me? I've heard similar stories, such as a recent newlywed with the post-wedding blues or the sports hero with a letdown after winning the championship game.

Your career can bring you the ultimate sense of accomplishment, but it can still leave a void that cannot be filled with adding more work. Trust me, I have tried. At one point I had two full-time jobs and a volunteer position! When you are looking for purpose, it often is not found by adding successes in the same area. That leaves you feeling more physically and mentally exhausted. Filling this space means taking a realistic look at yourself, at what truly satisfies you. You have to explore what brings your life true contentment. This means asking some pretty serious questions. *What excites me? What is important to me? What do I enjoy doing with my time?* These can be personal or professional aims, but at the end of the day, they must aid in providing a sense of purpose.

Some common areas that provide fulfillment beyond your current career are spiritual enlightenment, career change, improvement of or progression in relationships, motherhood, aiding those in need, traveling, and developing a hobby or skill. But this is by no means an exhaustive list. Your story is unique and your path distinctive. Without asking yourself the important questions to gain some direction, you may get stuck in that wrong pair of shoes!

WHAT DOES YOUR SUCCESS LOOK LIKE?

When I begin therapy with an individual or couple, I ask them to describe what the goal or expected outcome of their therapy is, to define what a successful therapy trial would look like. This reminds me to keep their objective in focus as we move forward so that we do not lose perspective. I am fascinated by the differences in aspirations and definitions of success I hear. So success is not the same for everyone. From massive amounts of money, to notoriety, to white picket fences, to spiritual growth, I've heard it all.

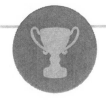

" It is important for you to know what success looks like for you."

It is important for you to know what success looks like for you. This cannot be based on the views and opinions of others or society. As a Modern Trophy Wife, you seek to enrich yourself and the world around you, but how you accomplish that is completely personalized. You have to decide what kind of person you want to be and what impact you want to have. What kind of things do you admire in others that might make you proud? When do you feel the most accomplished? Your definition of success may change along the way as you grow and develop, and that's fine. But if you do not stop periodically to think about what you value and what you are striving for, you may never achieve it.

STOP COMPARING YOURSELF TO OTHERS

Nowadays, you can witness the ins and outs of just about anyone's life. You can view pictures on social media, watch a video sent on Snapchat, or even tune in to a reality show of your favorite celebrity. But what do you really know his or her real story? We form opinions of others' lives from what we see or hear, all the while not knowing their full narrative. Or maybe you have the details. You know how much money they have or the things they have acquired. You've heard all about how amazing their jobs are. How great their husbands treat them. You feel a pang of jealousy because you hate your job, you can't remember your last date night, or you can barely afford to pay back your student loans.

One of the hardest things to do is to stop comparing yourself to others. It is like a reflex. You see yourself in relation to others because it is how you initially form an idea of being a person. Comparative thinking starts when we are children. We begin life as a blank slate and learn how to act by mimicking those around us. They mirror back whether a behavior is desired. Our caregivers slowly allow us to have more freedoms, to test our limits. We then leave home and are on our own. We learn even more about ourselves and the world. A major challenge in life is how we become mature in our thought process and form our own identity—what most people call a sense of self. But it remains difficult to hear our own voices and form our own conclusions when for so long we mimicked others and did what they told us. We were concerned about how others viewed us.

It is so easy to elicit only the information that you want to perceive. You see the aspects of others' lives that you appreciate, not the full story. You see her hot husband and adorable children, not the mother with cancer. You see her thin and shapely frame, not her dead-end job. You start to take snapshots of everyone's story and create an ideal, leaving out negative aspects. If you are not careful, continued social comparisons can cause self-esteem issues and lead to anxiety or depression. Social comparison has become more frequent in the digital age, with the ability to get a front-row seat at the show of information that people want to give.

Ladies, it is time to break the cycle of social comparison. All humans are created equal. Take away money, beauty, and the appearance of happiness, and you will see that all people have strengths and weaknesses, highs and lows, and insecurities. Having things or achieving goals does not make anyone immune from tragedy or mortality. You do not know anyone's internal struggles other than your own, so don't compare your worst to someone else's best! Don't get me wrong—you can be *inspired* by others. Comparing is evaluating or measuring yourself against others, whereas inspiration is looking to the outside for motivation or encouragement. Inspiration is a beautiful thing as it often leads to positive change or stimulation on the inside.

The only person you need to evaluate is the person you are today, to analyze whether you are moving in the right direction. Celebrate your own personal successes, and learn from your own mistakes. The more time you spend looking outward, the less time you have to look inward. Use your precious time to learn about and develop yourself.

Your journey is unique. Your story is your own.

Now go and live it!

DO MORE OF WHAT YOU LOVE

My friends often tease me for being a Zumba fanatic. I go multiple times a week regardless of what is going on in my life. "It's not an effective workout," they say. "You don't burn enough calories," they say. I constantly receive invitations to try different workouts or change my workout schedule. What they do not understand is that I do Zumba for fun! I love dancing to the music and learning new moves. For that one hour, I can step outside of my head and relax. I can truly enjoy myself without worrying about other people or my responsibilities. Have I tried barre fitness and HIIT? Yes! We can get swept up in fashion trends, fad diets, or other crazes, but at the end of the day, we have to return to what centers us. I will fit my Zumba in somewhere.

We often get caught up in doing what is expected of us or doing what we think other people want. Do you feel pressured to stay in a certain profession? Do you feel guilty for not wanting to have children right away? As I've mentioned, living for others or trying to maintain appearances usually leaves you exhausted and unfulfilled. You spend energy on things that don't satisfy your needs and are left empty. You live to please, impress, or pacify others, but at the end of the day, you do not feel good about yourself. Why should your needs come last?

Ladies, you need to regain control of your life and make more self-focused choices. Fill your days with more things that bring you joy. If you haven't found your "Zumba," you should search for it. Determine what activity or interest makes you content. I've seen individuals achieve bliss in traveling, painting, or writing, and a friend of mine delights in puzzles. Whatever you realize brings you to a happy place, where you can be carefree and catch yourself smiling—do that more often. This can be a profession, a hobby, or a passion. I once met a woman at the gym who was so excited to tell me that she was making specialized tutus and selling them online. I'm pretty sure there were naysayers who told her the tutu market was slim to none, but she sold so many orders she had to enlist the help of a friend to meet them all.

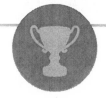

> **"Whatever you realize brings you to a happy place, where you can be carefree and catch yourself smiling— do that more often."**

I know what you're thinking: that you are already stuck in a situation, don't have enough time, or have too many obligations. You're in a dead-end career, your marriage has hit a rough patch, or your idea has never made it off the ground. But it is never too late to change the way your life is focused. As we discussed, there will always be an excuse to hold you back.

So ditch that corporate job and become a life coach. Set your first couple's therapy appointment. Delay that child for another year. Do *you*. Of course, there will be times that you have to do things you would rather not, or times you are not able to participate in something that moves you. But it is within your power to limit these occasions. It is time to start doing more of what you want, not what people or society makes you feel like you should want.

Focus on the Positive

Thoughts can be powerful. Research shows that the average person can have close to 50,000 thoughts in a day.[1] Self-talk is the flow of unspoken conversation or commentary in your head. Your inner voice says all of the things you don't say out loud. This talk is automatic, like a reflex, and is going on continuously. Sometimes, you don't even realize it is happening. These thoughts can be positive or negative, and they can have a profound impact on how you feel. With all of that action going on in our heads, it is no wonder that we can often lose sight of our overall vision. It is very important to understand our thoughts, as they affect our emotions, which in turn affect our behavior. What starts as one pessimistic idea can be the launching pad for a cascading of negative thoughts, feelings, and actions, an avalanche gaining momentum and leading to destruction in its path.

Do you find that you tend to replay or fixate on a negative idea or situation? Try as you might, you just can't seem to shake the thoughts regarding why something happened, what you should have done differently, or how someone else should have responded. You notice that afterward, your whole day seems to go poorly and nothing seems to be going right for you. Then comes a new wave of negative thoughts regarding how everything is horrible, and you can never catch a break. The more you try to tell yourself to stop thinking about things, the more you seem to obsess about it.

"The way to battle a negative thought is to flood it with positive ones."

This process is called rumination. Rumination is when you compulsively focus on the causes and symptoms of the issue, the upsetting aspects of a situation. This sort of thinking is not solution driven; it is cause oriented. Instead of looking forward and at possible problem solving, you get stuck on the reasons and consequences of the circumstance. This process can exhaust you mentally, emotionally, and physically; you are placing your energy in a futile direction.

People often think they have no control over the thoughts in their head, that they just happen. Well, I have some exciting news! There is a tested way to combat your negative thoughts and end the ruminative cycle. The solution is to shift the conversation in your head in a positive direction. In other words, the way to battle a negative thought is to flood it with positive ones.

Positive thinking does not mean that you ignore any negative things that come up; it simply means you redirect your focus to positive or productive aspects of a situation. It is about recognizing negative thoughts and challenging them with positive self-talk. Positive self-talk is being optimistic and encouraging toward yourself and your life situations. It is giving yourself the grace and understanding that you often give to others. This is the key to breaking the downward spiral of pessimism.

Here are some tips for how to start addressing negativity with positive thinking:

1. **Identify your ruminating negative thoughts**

   This is the first step in the process of becoming more positive. Identifying the discouraging and destructive things that you are telling yourself on a daily basis is necessary to change your patterns. Do you blame yourself when something bad happens? Do you ignore all of the positive things that happen in a situation and look only at the negative things? These are signs of negative thinking and areas where some positive thinking can intervene.

2. **Identify situations or people associated with negative emotions**

   If you can't immediately pinpoint your negative thoughts, it may be easier to look at specific situations or interactions that cause you worry or other negative emotions, such as meetings with certain colleagues, going to the gym, or visiting your in-laws. You likely have negative thoughts that run through your head when going into these situations, so pay more attention to what is leading to those negative feelings.

3. **Check in**

   Throughout your day, I want you to intermittently stop what you are doing and examine the content of your thoughts. Do they have a negative spin to them? Then think about how you are feeling. Are your feelings at all related to what you are thinking? Checking in can be a powerful tool in managing your thoughts before they get the best of you or control your mood and actions.

4. **Rehearse positive self-talk**

Once you recognize that your thoughts are negative or heading in a negative direction, respond with a positive thought or affirmation. Try to place a positive spin on any thought that seems negative, or think of a way you can be productive. If this does not seem to work, go with positive affirmations! Positive affirmations are statements that describe a desired situation or goal. When repeated regularly, they can lighten your mood and produce euphoric feelings. Try using affirmations after you check in and identify negative thoughts or emotions. You can even try repeating them at the start of your day to get in the right mindset!

Here are some of my favorite affirmations to get you started:

- *I am at peace.*
- *My thoughts are under my control.*
- *I am surrounded by love.*
- *I radiate love and happiness.*
- *I am healthy and happy.*
- *The more grateful I am, the more reasons I find to be grateful.*
- *When I believe in myself, so do others.*
- *I am my own unique self—original, inspired, and amazing.*
- *I trust in the process of life.*
- *I choose love, joy, and freedom.*
- *My heart is open and allows wonderful things to flow into my life.*

Applying these steps will help you learn to break the pattern of negative thoughts and consequently, negative emotions and behaviors. You will likely start seeing more positive results in how you feel about yourself and your life. Get started today!

Notes

CHAPTER

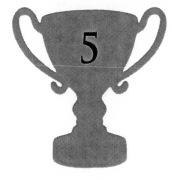

5

"The secret of success is seeing the value in every moment."

THE MODERN TROPHY WIFE MANAGES TIME EFFECTIVELY

My time is now precious. As I told you in chapter 2, my time was "semi-valuable" in my twenties. Every now and then, I would go to events I wasn't really interested in or hang out with others for something to do rather than really wanting to be in their company. As I mentioned, the value of my time has skyrocketed in my thirties to being pretty darn close to priceless. The balance of a full-time career, motherhood, marriage, and fitness is not a cakewalk. It's more of a tightrope balancing act. It's important to remain standing in all these areas to manage your time effectively. Things go downhill pretty fast once you get off balance. As Modern Trophy Wives, we have too many important things on our plates to take the risk of everything tumbling down.

THE PITFALLS OF OVERSCHEDULING

Let's start by addressing the pitfalls of poor time management. I'm sure we all have been culprits of this at one time in our calendars. You put too much on the to-do list and you end up bone tired. You know what happens when a Modern Trophy Wife becomes exhausted? These bad emotions can quickly rear their head:

Sad, snappy, and sleepless

These are the dreaded *S*'s that can pop into the future of overscheduled wives. They are grouped together because they often come as a trio. All three might not happen at once, but their arrival times are usually pretty close. Your mood is usually the first to suffer. Women who spread themselves too thin can experience increased irritability, feelings of sadness, and sometimes hopelessness that things won't get better. It affects not only you but your family as well. Your husband may notice the second *S* first, where you are more likely to snap over things that you wouldn't normally mind. You are easily annoyed, and your household feels the aftershock of your short temper. Some may even run for cover! You know the quote "Happy Wife, Happy Life"? This concept is what that quote is based on. If the wife isn't happy, no one is.

"Your mood is usually the first to suffer."

In my practice, I have seen women who are so exhausted that they have experienced muscle tightness, poor concentration, and just a general feeling of being on edge. These are all classic symptoms of anxiety. Some women can experience more severe anxiety, resulting in actual panic attacks. These can consist of problems breathing and chest pains and even feel as severe as a heart attack. All these mood symptoms are not to be taken lightly. They are symptoms of stress. The more stress you have, the weaker your immune system can become. This opens the door for you to be more susceptible to chronic illnesses such as heart disease, high blood pressure, and digestive problems.

The next thing that usually gets sacrificed when women overschedule is sleep. From the medical standpoint, this is one of the worst things that you can give up. You have already heard me mention the benefits of a good night's rest. When you start sleeping less to get everything done, it becomes a vicious cycle. You are now sleep deprived, which can make you more anxious and depressed. Because your schedule is bursting at the seams, you have no time to catch up on the sleep you need. Something's gotta give. You cannot carry on this way. Another potential roadblock is when you actually want to sleep but can't get the sleep you need. You have problems falling asleep, you wake up multiple times throughout the night, or you wake up too early in the mornings. Just as poor sleep can lead to feeling stressed, the converse is true as well. Anxiety, mental exhaustion, and sadness can lead to problems falling asleep. I have seen women turn to sleeping medications or alcohol to help remedy the problem. This actually can make things worse, leading to drug or alcohol abuse problems pretty quickly.

Ladies, we need our beauty rest. It's not just for our outer beauty but for the inner beauty also. Anxiety and sadness are common results of an overly packed schedule. If you're not sure if you qualify as overscheduled, take a look at your calendar and do regular mood checks. You will soon figure it out.

Resentful

When you give too much to others, you sometimes can develop feelings of resentment. Women have revealed to me that they began to resent their kids and/or husband due to giving so much to them and so little to themselves. They are often very ashamed of having such ill feelings toward their family and only reveal it to me as their doctor. However, it's not something to be ashamed of. Resentment is a result of us overextending ourselves and can linger a long time if not addressed.

The first step in addressing resentment is recognizing the feelings and what has caused them. Often, the people don't even know you resent them because you are the one who so generously offered your time. Now, I am not saying you let them know your feelings of resentment. A phone call or text stating "I resent you" won't be received too well on the other end. However, you should recognize why you may be feeling resentful and what changes can be made to relieve that. These changes usually involve stepping back a little and asking for help when you need it or simply saying no.

Mentally exhausted

We already discussed what happens with a tired body, but being mentally drained can wreak just as much havoc. You often don't have the energy to pursue the things that make you happy, including the so-important self-care. As humans, we automatically put in less effort when we are fatigued. This means that work projects, date nights, and meals cooked for your family don't get your full attention. They become subpar. I know that when I am mentally exhausted, I specifically neglect working on my dream goals. When I am trying to stay above water, working toward my destiny suddenly gets pushed to the back of the to-do pile. That is a huge wake-up call for me.

" Be wise in where you deposit your efforts."

You have to protect your emotional energy and realize that you only have a reserved supply. Be wise in where you deposit your efforts. You cannot say yes to everything. You must steer clear of anything that involves extra drama because that will deplete your emotional stores twice as fast. We have enough crises and obstacles that can happen naturally in life. For that very reason, I advise you to make an effort to avoid those who like to create conflict with others or make major problems out of small things. They do nothing but wear you out.

TIPS TO GET MORE OUT OF YOUR TIME

Just say no

No is one of the shortest words in our vocabulary yet the most difficult for us to say. It doesn't help that with today's technology, people can contact you in a gazillion different ways to ask you to do something. My most common mode of communication for receiving requests is text. I figure it's because people would rather hear a *no* via text instead of in person or on the phone. Somehow, it makes the refusal seem less harsh to both the giver and the receiver.

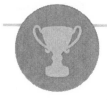

> **" It makes life simpler and also contributes to a happier marriage when you do things you actually want to do."**

My rule of thumb for considering a request is to ask yourself two questions first: Can I do it (time- and energy-wise) and, just as important in my book (pun intended), do I really want to do it? When I get a text request, I literally stare at the phone for a good ten seconds before I respond, contemplating the two questions above. If I answer no to either of my questions, a text saying no is sent and case closed.

People often spend more time laboring over what excuse to give or even worse, they give in and say yes out of guilt. The guilt-filled *yes* guarantees that you will have a miserable experience. The key is to say no and say it quickly. It is often a reflex that if saying no, we must give at least one valid excuse to accompany our answer. That is not necessary.

I watched a recent interview with Shonda Rhimes and Oprah Winfrey in which Shonda discussed how she began saying no to things she didn't want to do. She noticed incredible results in how much happier she became. Instead of giving elaborate reasons for her *no*, she just said, "No, I'm not able to do that." That's it. That's gold! It's polite and to the point. My advice is to use this phrase or one similar in your denials. It's best to say no in the most efficient yet courteous way possible.

Remember, stay strong. Those guilt trips can have some pretty gusty winds after a *no*, but keep your feet mounted on the ground. Do not give in. It makes life simpler and also contributes to a happier marriage when you do things you actually want to do.

Prioritize

A key to getting a handle on your schedule is to prioritize your activities. I always make sure the most important things get placed at the top of the list. The top is filled with things that need to be done for me to function at my best. My weekday list includes morning prayer, going to the gym before work, addressing any urgent hubby/kid needs, and giving the best care to my patients. These are the core activities of my day, and then I plan the rest of my day accordingly.

Other list items that should be considered for the top may also include all forms of self-care, speaking with loved ones, and making time each day to work toward your dream goals. Once you prioritize, it's easier to fill that schedule based on what serves you the best. What is on your list of core activities that you have to get done daily? Do you participate in any activities now that aren't necessary or don't really provide any benefit?

"Don't underestimate the power of being still."

In addition to evaluating what should be at the top of your list, you also need to look at what can be taken off the list. Do you have a thirty-minute conversation with a coworker every day that isn't very fulfilling or even interesting? Shorten that exchange and start doing something you would rather do. Fill that time with looking up a restaurant for the next girls' dinner, text your husband something romantic, or how about just be still and meditate? I know for you career wives and especially for you mothers that peace is something to be treasured. It is often few and far between in your hectic lives. Don't underestimate the power of being still. Even just five to ten minutes of doing nothing can be quite rejuvenating. Try it tomorrow.

Get a grasp on social media

In terms of priorities, this is a good time to see where social media ranks on your list. With easy access from our phones and computers, a few minutes of a glance at a profile can quickly snowball into more than an hour daily of scrolling through pictures and reading comments. Americans in all walks of life are spending hours a day on social media sites.[2] Is that the best use of your time? If you find it to be a stress reliever, then by all means carry on. However, if you find it as more of a distraction, consider stepping away from the screen.

There have been studies of people who noticed that they felt worse after scrolling through their social media timelines. Not having regular face-to-face contact can lead to people having feelings of loneliness rather than the connectedness they desire. Also, many describe a "FOMO" (feeling of missing out) when looking at friends' pictures. They may have feelings of envy and inadequacy when they see friends flaunt a luxurious or adventurous lifestyle. If scrolling takes up a lot of time and makes you feel bad, just stop.

Social media can also become a hazard in marriages. I have seen marriages enter rough waters from connections made online. Some of these couples were able to find their way back to safe land, and some ended in the abyss of divorce. With that said, be very careful with how you play the social media game. It's just natural that people are more likely to flirt online than in person. Also, beware of exes popping up in the "People You May Know" column. I actually think this should come with a flashing *Danger* sign when you click on it.

Some of you ladies reading right now might think I'm overreacting, because what's the harm in liking a few pictures or having casual conversation online? I have seen the aftereffects of this lead to jealousy, mistrust, and sometimes the end of marriages. Tread lightly!

The next time you're cruising your News Feed, check your watch. Are those minutes (or hours) spent on social media contributing something positive to your day? As a Modern Trophy Wife, you must watch out for activities that can suck your time without providing any real benefit. You have so much more you could be doing instead.

FIGHT PROCRASTINATION

You have prioritized your agenda and your schedule is now filled with items you want to do. However, you've noticed that you don't feel like starting that project at the top of your list. This is how procrastination starts, and it can be the kryptonite to Modern Trophy Wives. Procrastinators wait until they "feel like" doing an action. The issue is that the motivated feeling hardly ever comes on its own. Procrastinators find everything else in the world to distract themselves from doing what they need to do.

I can speak from experience. In college, I quickly learned about the pitfalls of procrastinating. If I didn't start writing my English literature paper after class in the evening, by midnight I definitely didn't want to write it. I had convinced myself that if I cleaned my room, chatted on AOL, took a nap, and watched just one episode of *Frasier* that somehow I would get a surge of energy to write a paper about nineteenth-century poetry in the middle of the night. It took a few "not so great" grades following pretty awful papers written in the wee hours of the morning for me to realize that procrastination was evil. I started working on my assignments earlier and spread them out over several days rather than several hours. My grades improved, and I was able to sleep a decent night before the due date without having the 1 a.m. feeling of doom that my paper wouldn't be done in time.

We are really psyching ourselves out by procrastinating because we're making ourselves dread it even more by putting it off. As a Modern Trophy Wife, we have too much on our plates to let procrastination get in the way. The key is to just get started and get the engine running. Once you start, you will soon realize the task isn't the ordeal that you imagined. The more you get done, the more motivated you are to complete the next step.

Here are some practical tips to battle procrastination:

1. **Set a schedule for yourself where you break down projects into small tasks**

   For example, you have been traveling for work, meeting deadlines, and also going on couple's date nights with your husband. Your walk-in closet is now a disaster area. It's turned into a pile of work slacks, pajamas, heels, and suitcases. You know it will take about four hours to clean your closet, including taking out clothes you don't wear anymore and organizing what you do wear. My advice is to break up the project into manageable parts. Break it in half so that you do a couple of hours today and a couple hours tomorrow. You can even break it into smaller increments in which you do an hour a day for four days. Monday, you organize your pants, Tuesday, you can organize your shoes, and so on.

This technique has worked wonders for me to get things done. My most effective approach is working in smaller increments over a longer span of time. Somehow, knowing that I don't have to complete it all in one day makes the task less daunting, and I can get it done more efficiently.

2. Write down the disadvantages of procrastinating

Once again, my putting-pen-to-paper rule comes to light. I want you to write down some bad things that may happen if you keep waiting to get started. For the closet task, some disadvantages could include having to look at a messy closet daily, longer times to find your clothes to get dressed in the morning, and creating a tripping hazard with your shoes all over the place. When you sit down to really consider the disadvantages of procrastinating on your particular task, this might give you the nudge you need to make that first move.[3]

3. Don't be afraid to ask for help to get started

I love to travel and I love to pack. However, I truly dislike unpacking (which leads to the messy closet scenario). I will confess that I have returned from a trip and my suitcase has stayed on my bedroom floor for more than a week. My procrastination has been so bad that if I've needed to wear something in the suitcase, I will just retrieve that one item instead of unpacking it all. I have come to terms with this and I know it's something on my procrastination list. What do I do? I call for backup. I ask my dear husband to unpack with me. We unpack the day after our return home, and we do it together. I get it done much more efficiently when he unpacks his suitcase alongside me. In hindsight, I should have asked for help with this years ago. It would have prevented a few stubbed toes on suitcases in the middle of the night. This is a simple example, but it can be applied to many different types of tasks.

4. **Never stop focusing on the light at the end of the tunnel**

   In medical school, we had test blocks in which basically all of our tests for every subject always fell within the same week. It was easy to fall in the rabbit hole of being overwhelmed. Focusing on what I was going to do after the tests is one of the things that kept me going. After taking our epic posttest naps, we would celebrate by going out to eat, going dancing, or just hanging out with friends. Dr. Gathing and I had some pretty noteworthy celebrations after those tests. Those nights were magical, and I was always looking forward to the next one. This helped me not to procrastinate and kept my eyes on the prize. If I could get through that week, then the celebration would be that much sweeter.

   Whatever your light at the end of the tunnel may be after accomplishing your task list, never lose sight. It's going to keep your motor running.

5. **Take social media apps off your phone temporarily**

   It's a quick and effective strategy. Once you're done, feel free to add them back. Remember, social media and procrastination go hand in hand. They're like besties: where one is, you will find the other. Avoid them both.

BETTER TIME MANAGEMENT = BETTER YOU

More "me time"

The more you get done in a timely fashion, the more time you have to unwind. You are not in relaxation mode if you're thinking about all the things that didn't get done. That is called guilt, and it can ruin a rest day in an instant. When you manage your time well, guilt is no longer a factor because you know you made the best use of your time. You know that you deserve a break. Always keep in mind that a rest stop is up ahead as you go through your week of tasks and events. Your personal respite is one of the many rewards of effective time management. If you can't figure out what to do during your break, refer back to chapter 1 about self-care.

Improved time management equals more rest for you in the long run. A rested Modern Trophy Wife is a happy one.

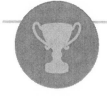

> **"You are not in relaxation mode if you're thinking about all the things that didn't get done."**

The more efficient you are, the happier you are

Efficiency in your daily life boosts your sense of accomplishment and self-esteem. It's a simple cause and effect. It makes you feel good about getting things done at home and at work. You are no longer running out of control on the treadmill of life. You have now mastered a way to keep a steady tempo at the pace that works best for you. At the end of each week, reflect on what you've accomplished. You will be stunned by how many things got done. Sometimes, I actually count all the things I have crossed off my list. I realize I'm a star and give myself credit for a job well done. This may seem too self-gratifying to some of you wives. As Modern Trophy Wives, however, there is absolutely nothing wrong with patting ourselves on the back. All positive reinforcement is good, even if it's coming from ourselves. We have to recognize that we are winning.

Happy wife, happy life (happy husband, happy kids, happy family)

It is a fact that your relationships can improve when you feel you have your life more under control. When you have designated times to devote to the people most important to you, it leads to your loved ones feeling valued. The more valued they feel, the more likely they are to reciprocate. This can dramatically improve the dynamic of a relationship, especially with loved ones who may have felt neglected with your busy schedule in the past. Your support network is just as vital to your success. Your time management with the inclusion of time spent with them leads to more support and further success.

Your time is precious. Once you fully grasp that, you will begin shifting your life to match its value. The main points I want you to remember are to be cognizant of what you say yes to, schedule with priority, and fight the procrastination evil. Overall, these three principles are essential to getting what you need out of your days.

There are many tempting distractions in this world, and at times, those diversions will try to take you off course. Distractions can be anything ranging from dramatic friends, social media, gossip, and other bad habits. The tools of effective time management will help keep you on track in your many roles. It will keep you healthy, help your relationships thrive, and help you accomplish your goals. The first step in practicing effective time management is placing value on your time. Once you value something, you make better decisions on where your time is spent. This practice will not only keep your feet on the ground but also propel you to fly to higher levels. You have too big of a destiny to fulfill to be wasting time.

Notes

CHAPTER

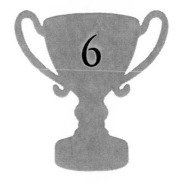

6

"You can reach for the sky because you have a strong support system."

THE MODERN TROPHY WIFE BUILDS STRONG RELATIONSHIPS

I have learned a great deal from working with individuals and families, but I would say the most important thing I've realized is that success is rarely attained alone. A key to reaching your goals and maintaining your sanity is to have a network of strong relationships helping you along the way. When I hear success stories in my field, they tout a spiritual foundation, a friend network, or an involved mentor. In essence, I hear a sense of community. The community is made up of special people behind the scenes making it all possible. The real MVPs.

As someone who is constantly striving to enrich yourself and the world, you have taken on a number of roles and responsibilities. You have a number of people in your life who care about and depend on you. But who do you depend on? Who provides support for you?

You are doing it wrong by trying to be some kind of Superwoman. Doing it all on your own does not make you Superwoman; it just makes you super tired! You are already a boss, wife, mommy, volunteer, leader, and friend to many. Each day, you wake up and face the world full steam ahead, but at the end of your day, you are empty. When was the last time you phoned a friend and discussed how exhausted you sometimes feel? Dropped your kids off at a friend's to have a date night with your hubby?

Or had your coworker cover while you took a long vacation from work responsibilities? And I don't mean the kind of vacation where you are still checking your email or putting out fires so you don't have to deal with them later.

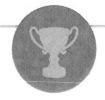

"Doing it all on your own does not make you Superwoman; it just makes you super tired!"

Ladies, it is time for you to develop and make use of a network of supports as you strive to achieve your dreams. Building a strong support system is about creating connections, nurturing the relationships, and providing give and take. Having this system allows you to balance your daily activities with your journey to greatness.

Let's discuss the concept of cultivating strong relationships to get you through the best and worst of times.

TEAMWORK MAKES THE DREAM WORK

Social support is providing care, assistance, and resources to others, usually friends and loved ones. Social support can come in various forms, but most important are emotional and instrumental aid. Emotional support can be the most beneficial aspect of having strong relationships. It includes the actions others take to make you feel cared for. When receiving emotional support, you have a safe place to share your feelings and be truthful without judgment. It provides a sense of security when times are rough. Instrumental support is physical aid such as monetary, transportation, or childcare. Soliciting this type of support can be difficult. You feel that you cannot ask for or do not need help from those around you, despite giving such support to others. You give but don't take.

Research has shown that social support wards off the effects of a number of health problems, including depression and anxiety.[4] However, many of us are not connected with others or do not regularly use the network we have. In today's society, there is less of a sense of community than ever before. Many of us do not even know our neighbors! We are less focused on building relationships with others and have not strengthened the ones we do have because we are too focused on our daily grind. You may have five hundred Facebook friends but only one or two actual friends you can count on when the chips are down. You have to do better!

It is not as easy as it once was to meet people with similar interests and maintain closeness. In an era where social networking is at an all-time high, surveys show that connectedness is at an all-time low. I'm not saying social media is a negative thing, especially when reaching those who may be geographically distant. However, to develop true bonds that build strong supports, you must put in the work, time, and energy. Once formed, these relationships can offer the stability you need to progress in all areas of your life.

It is imperative that you use your network to provide the support you need to achieve your potential. There is no "who can do everything themselves" contest, so you do not have to be a martyr. If you're not convinced, here are some of the many benefits of building and using a support network:

1. **A sense of connection**

   Having a close network of supports can provide a sense of belonging and prevent isolation. Being around like-minded individuals delivers instant access to advice, information, and, in some cases, commiseration. It reminds you that you are not alone in a world full of chaos. It is reassuring to know that you have people there if you ever need a listening ear. Or maybe just someone to laugh with! Sometimes you just need to be around folks you can be yourself with. It also doesn't hurt that they often remind you of how wonderful you are and toot your horn. Ladies, you need that encouragement every now and then to remember how amazing you are.

2. **Stress reduction**

   It is well documented that social support is a coping mechanism that leads to significant reductions in stress.[5] When we see our friends and close loved ones, we experience a rise in neurotransmitters and hormones that make us feel good. This in turn decreases the presence of negative emotions and stress. Girls' night out can literally make it all better! Receiving emotional and tangible support when juggling your responsibilities leads to stress reduction by diminishing role conflicts. In other words, when you have someone to lean on in times of need, it reduces issues with competing roles and priorities. Calling a friend to babysit or having your parent make a cake for the bake sale can relieve a sense of desperation. And you do not have to feel guilty about it! You can also use your network to problem solve and manage difficult situations. Your connections may have some input or be able to jump in and lend a hand. Take that hand!

3. **Resilience**

Resilience is the ability to adapt well when confronted with difficult or trying situations. You are resilient when you are able to face and conquer adversity. Having strong relationships and supports is a known protective factor when dealing with misfortune. When dealing with tragedy or traumatic events, from financial difficulties to severe illness, you are more likely to rebound and get back to a stable place when you have people in your corner. Your network can provide encouragement, resources, supervision, and direction as needed. Having support has been shown to enhance immune function and increase endorphins, making you more likely to manage stress, survive illness, and tolerate pain.[6] In fact, studies in cancer, Alzheimer's, and cardiovascular disease show a better prognosis and survival rate for patients with strong and active support systems.[7] This is also true with depression, anxiety, and schizophrenia. Our confidants are literally lifesavers!

#SquadGoals

Now you are convinced. You see the benefits of strong relationships and want to explore this further, but you don't have a support system. Maybe you've alienated your friends with your constant business; moved away from family to get some space; or like to keep it casual with coworkers. It is not unusual for a completely likable and fun woman to find herself without a circle. Your closet buddies have spread across the country in search of love and success, and the encounters you have with other women seem superficial or lacking common interests. Or maybe you do not get out much or meet new people at all because you are an introvert.

It is easy to find peers who want to go out and party or attend the latest social event, but it is much more difficult to make quality contacts with a similar mindset. You are looking to meet women who also want to enrich their lives and nurture their families but know how to kick back and have a good time, too. You know how to enjoy yourself and have already had your share of parties, but you are now more focused on self-care and growth than shutting down the club. You want to engage with other women who share these interests, not women who are one-dimensional, like those solely focused on entertainment or activities surrounding wifehood or motherhood. You want to be in the company of other women who see themselves as a work in progress, who are constantly striving for self-improvement.

So how do you build a support system when you can barely maintain the life you have? Here are some options you can tap into in order to build positive connections:

1. **Connect with acquaintances**

   This may be the simplest way to establish a network. You have likely encountered acquaintances over time but never thought to follow up with them. These may be friends of friends, known by loved ones, or known through work connections. If you think for a second, you will recall someone you have come across who seemed genuine and shared common interests. You both may have been new wives, new mothers, pet owners, or in the same industry. You seemed to click at the time, but with the hustle and bustle of life, you didn't really give it a second thought.

   Or maybe you were a part of a group of friends and didn't spend much time with someone but could now reach out to reconnect. Don't forget that you can also reach out to old friends you might have lost touch with over time. These women may have also led busy lives that led to the relationship fizzling out, but they may be open to reconnecting.

2. **Join a gym or active group**

I am no gym rat by any means, but I do recognize the benefits of exercise. We have already explored the effects exercise has on your well-being, but it can also have a profound effect on your social network. The gym is a place where women of all types from all walks of life congregate. You may not socialize very much if you are there now, but that can change. I was never the type to speak to people or strike up conversations at the gym, but after moving to a new city and knowing no one, I ended up talking to a woman who also loved Zumba. We exchanged numbers and became fast friends. She became my accountability partner, friend, and eventually my new Zumba teacher! She has been there along the way helping to motivate me, problem solve, and keep it real.

Numerous women out there may be looking for new connections and willing to partner up for the buddy system. You may be able to help each other out in your workouts and perhaps provide accountability. Doing workouts you enjoy will offer entertainment while in a setting where you can also get to know each other better. These workouts can include recreation groups such as running, hiking, or biking groups as well as team sports such as kickball or volleyball.

3. **Explore your hobby**

As discussed, it is always great to spend time doing the things you enjoy. If you have a hobby you can perform while meeting others, that is even better. Often, there are hobbies you can do alone but with options to make them social, such as cooking classes, wine tastings, or salsa classes. The new wine-and-paint craze has been a great way to mingle and meet new people while creating works of art. Breaking out of your shell and participating in a class or group can not only introduce you to more people but also allow you to learn new things or share ideas and information.

4. Start online networking

Ladies, here is where you can make the Internet work for you. Instead of cyberstalking and catching up on celebrity gossip, you can
use the Internet and social media to move from the digital world to
an actual social one. Online networking is an amazing opportunity
to bring people together.

Once I settled in my new city five years ago, I rebuilt a network
from joining a Meetup group for young professional women. I met
women with similar backgrounds who were also looking to connect,
and I am still friends with them to this day. There are other online
social networking sites that can connect you with women who have
common interests. You just have to run an online search and keep
an open mind! Not only can you use these groups to meet others,
but you can also use them for ideas of places to go and explore.

Using online resources, you can also discover local networking
events, which are great places to meet new people. These events
can revolve around certain industries, social events, or professional
organizations. They are a great way to meet new people who interest you as well as open yourself up to new opportunities to enrich
yourself in the process.

5. Go to church

Church is a place for spiritual growth and enlightenment, a place
where you can become closer to God. But church can also be a place
where you become closer to other believers and build a network.
Churches frequently hold Bible studies and small group activities,
as well as provide ministries for members with various interests.
They also have seminars and conferences tailored to meet the needs
of certain groups, such as women, men, singles, married couples,
and senior citizens. Most events have childcare and teachers readily
available and assigned to watch your children while you focus on
learning and worshipping.

Many churches have websites and even downloadable appli-
cations that track social events and opportunities for you to come
together with like-minded individuals. Whether you are taking part
in a ministry, joining a small group, or attending Bible study, you

will be sure to encounter others who want to grow their network or connect with new people.

6. **Join a support group**

One way to gain an instant network is to join a support group. This is different from building personal relationships as you are able to interact with multiple people in a group. Support groups are formed around a similar role, such as cancer survivors, caregivers of parents with Alzheimer's, trauma victims, family members of someone with a mental illness, or those with a history of substance use. These groups center on providing support, encouragement, advice, and shared experience. You may also form individual relationships within the group, and from there form a social network.

If you are dealing with a role that has been overwhelming for you, joining a support group may provide the sense of community that you need. You may gain access to tips, guidance, and tools that you can use in your daily life.

THE GOLDEN RULE

When was the last time you called up your friend to ask for help or assistance in some way? When was the last time you picked up the phone to call your friend (not text) and see how she was doing? Or, even more unlikely, when was the last time you offered to do something nice for someone without being prompted or expecting something in return? Be honest. While there is no shame in using your network and support system appropriately, you must also provide the same care and assistance in return. It is not often that we think about reciprocity within our relationships, as it normally comes naturally. You give a little, you take a little. You treat people the way that you want to be treated.

But in some cases, there becomes a one-sidedness to relationships. Someone does more of the giving or more of the taking, and that can become unhealthy. However, when both parties are invested and feel that the relationship is important, they will provide emotional and tangible support as necessary. When you look at your relationships, do you feel that they have an appropriate balance of give and take? This can be evaluated by ensuring that you respect each other's boundaries, provide emotional support, and give tangible assistance when able; you know you can trust one another with your feelings and information. How many of your relationships have a healthy balance, have reciprocity?

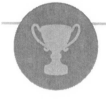

> **" It is time to invest in relationships that invest back into you, that pour into people who pour back into you."**

Ladies, it is time to manage your support network. It is time to invest in relationships that invest back into you, that pour into people who pour back into you. No more giving without taking and being left empty. And if you are the one who is constantly taking without giving in return, it is time to progress and start providing reciprocation. Live by the Golden Rule and treat others the way you want to be treated. This applies to all of your relationships—friends, coworkers, significant others, and other loved ones.

Once you have developed relationships, the way to foster them and create a lasting commitment is to nurture them and provide reciprocity. This creates the foundation for a lifelong connection of strong relationships and support for you as you achieve your life goals.

Male Supports

I am sure you are wondering why this chapter has not mentioned the support that you may receive from males. It has been primarily focused on support from other women. That's because when you become a wife or mother, there is a benefit in shared experience, of having someone who knows exactly what you may be going through or feeling. Men do not know the expectations that come with being a wife, mother, sister, and daughter, the constant conflict of being driven to nurture but needing to care for oneself. And as far as technology has come, men still do not have the ability to know what it is like to carry and birth a child, or all the physical and emotional havoc that comes with it.

But you may have a husband, brother, father, or friend you regularly turn to in times of need. They can provide tangible assistance, emotional support, and a social network, and they can give you that real opinion about your situation when you need it. This can be especially important when raising a child, as children of both sexes need male role models and benefit from having male supports in their life.

I have a loving husband, many male friends, and male family members I care about who provide support for me. My husband in particular is my biggest supporter, confidant, and best friend. He is constantly looking to make my life easier and better. I achieve the things I do and am able to strive for greatness because he is there with me along the way. Some of my other male supports I have known all my life or since I was a teenager, and they play a role in my well-rounded support system and network.

As a wife, it is important to let your husband know how to provide support to you. You may want him to be more affirming and let you know how he feels about you and the relationship. You may want him to help more around the house and with the children. Or you may want him to be more romantic and spontaneous, to take initiative in planning activities that promote bonding within your relationship.

No matter what, it takes you teaching your husband what supporting you looks like. Every person, every woman, is different, so he needs to know how to be more in tune with your needs. Do not make him guess what type of support may be the most helpful to you or what may relax you. Educating your husband on what relieves your stress or pours into your cup can be a big part of building your support system. It would be great if our husbands were psychic or could read us like a book! Instead of waiting on that miracle, how about just being open and honest about your desires? Let him know that even though you are strong, you do need him and value his assistance. Even if you think you could do it without him, why would you?

Now, ladies, a major part of using your husband as a support is that you do not criticize how he does things. You cannot be annoyed with the outfits he chooses for the children or that the meal he makes for the family is not nutritious enough. You cannot redo the cleaning that he did, or refold the clothes your way. Being overly critical of the support he provides when trying to assist you will lead to insecurity. He will feel like he should not try, as if he cannot live up to your standards. Your allowing him do things his way allows *you* to rest and have free time. Will your kids survive in a mismatched outfit? Yes. Will your kids develop heart problems from Daddy's no-veggies dinners? No. He loves your children and wants the best for them and you, so let him take care of you guys sometimes his way.

If you do have a husband or other male supports, that is wonderful. You should use that network to its full advantage. You may even learn a little something that the ladies haven't taught you!

IT TAKES A VILLAGE

Raising a child can be the most difficult role that you ever come across as a Modern Trophy Wife. It is a beautiful experience that can be exciting and rewarding. However, there is another side of parenting, a daunting reality that is faced on a regular basis. There are so many things people do not speak of when discussing parenthood, even with their closest confidants. The desperate thoughts you have when exhausted, the negative feelings you have toward your child at times, the hopelessness you feel because you don't feel in control. For those mothers who have postpartum depression or severe anxiety, these struggles can be even more pronounced. You are not alone.

When parents have a strong support network, they have improved outcomes and rate healthier in terms of well-being. But this network is not always easy to create. As previously discussed, you may not be in a position of having strong supports when you begin your journey into parenthood. You may live miles from family and have a network of friends without children. If you are in the minority of those who plan exactly when they want to start a family and have created a scenario where supports are readily available, then you are in good shape. But if you are like the vast majority and don't know the exact timing of things, you may be left scrambling before or after childbirth to create your village.

New responsibilities such as how to lay your child down at night to what type of school you should enroll your child in—there are so many things to decide and do. In my experience, parents who attempt to do these things without seeking support or guidance report lower emotional gratification from raising a child. So when you hear about the mom groups that meet up at the park and share their frustrations and joys, maybe you shouldn't laugh. When you hear about the couples who move to some little town to be closer to family, do not feel sorry for them. And when your in-laws suggest moving to your city, maybe you should rethink that instant *no*. Having a healthy number of supports close by to provide you relief, guidance, and assistance doesn't solve all the difficulties of parenting, but it sure makes it doable.

Once you have your network of support securely in place, figure out how best to use it. Do you want to have more time to work on personal goals or hobbies? Do you want to have more energy to put into your career? Do you want to have more girls' nights out? Whatever you decide, make sure that you use this added network to go for what you want and know that things will be okay.

" **Having a healthy number of supports close by to provide you relief, guidance, and assistance doesn't solve all the difficulties of parenting, but it sure makes it doable.** "

Notes

CHAPTER

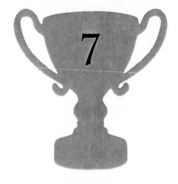

7

"Be a light that ignites passion in others."

THE MODERN TROPHY WIFE IS A ROLE MODEL AND MENTOR

The relationships you develop over time are priceless. As discussed in chapter 6, developing a network of like-minded individuals is essential to creating the balance required to pursue your dreams. Your confidants are used as resources and sounding boards, and at times they provide guidance in your day-to-day quandaries. These relationships provide the support you need to progress in your goals.

As your ambitions and purpose grow, you need to expand your circle to include connections who provide instruction and advice. The mentor-mentee relationship is an important step in your journey to achievement. As a Modern Trophy Wife, you recognize that there is always more to learn and more opportunities to evolve. (After all, you are reading this book because you are not a person who settles for mediocrity!) You may just need the right person asking you the tough questions or providing encouragement to make that next move.

Having a mentor who provides some direction and perspective along the way is vital to progression and achieving those challenging goals. Once you have explored and used the lessons a mentor has imparted, you are equipped to pass that experience on to someone else in need of guidance. Your unique talents blended with the knowledge gained from your mentor-mentee relationship allow you to become a leader and role model in your home and in the community.

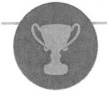

> " **As a Modern Trophy Wife, you recognize that there is always more to learn and more opportunities to evolve.**"

THE MENTOR-MENTEE RELATIONSHIP

Your life will constantly change, as will your advisory needs. Having someone in your life who is committed to assisting you reach your goals is indispensable. The reality is, you will likely have a number of people in your lifetime who aid in your development. You may seek out mentors for direction in your personal, career, and spiritual life, or you may even find someone who embodies all the areas in which you need guidance. You may be stuck in a personal rut, at a crossroads in your career, or looking for spiritual development. Or you may be in a good position in your life, but striving to achieve more ambitious goals.

You may not know where to begin in your search for a mentor. Or maybe you have a mentor in your life but do not feel that it is has been a very beneficial relationship. Here are some tips on how to get the most out of your mentor experiences:

1. **Make the right choice**
   Choosing the right individual to serve as your mentor is the key to getting the most out of the relationship. Identifying someone you admire is one part, but the other is choosing a person who has taken an active interest in your professional, personal, and/or spiritual growth. There is nothing more frustrating than selecting a mentor who does not have the time or is not willing to give the attention to your development that you deserve. Make sure you don't just choose the most knowledgeable or glamorous mentor but one who is truly invested in your future.

2. **Communicate your needs**

   Once you choose the right mentor, it is important that you are up-front about your expectations. It may be intimidating as this person is your role model, but you have to communicate your needs early on in the relationship. This may mean discussing his or her role in helping you reach your goals, the time commitment you expect, and any feedback you are soliciting. Develop a list of your desires for the mentor-mentee relationship and use it as a basis for your discussion.

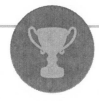

> " Having someone in your life who is committed to assisting you reach your goals is indispensable."

3. **Identify any resources or associates for connection**

   After building trust within the relationship, you can also approach your mentor for aid in expanding your personal or professional network. If your mentor is well connected, he or she can serve as a resource as well as an advocate for you. If you are honest about your goal of broadening your network, your mentor will likely introduce you to beneficial individuals. Be careful not to take advantage of or exploit these relationships.

4. **Welcome and accept constructive criticism**

   It is never easy to hear negative reviews about yourself, but constructive criticism is crucial to personal and professional development. If you never look at yourself with a critical eye, you will have difficulty knowing what areas to improve and sharpen. Your mentor can be the perfect person to deliver constructive criticism, as he or she is one of the few people in your life who can be objective. Handle the information with grace and apply the feedback where it is applicable.

5. **Ask the right questions**

   One of the best things about having a mentor is direct access to a wealth of knowledge in the area where you are hoping to thrive. Your mentor should be someone who has succeeded in your areas of interest. Whether looking to someone who has attained the personal life you are looking to or someone who has achieved your career goals, you will benefit from the knowledge of someone who has been where you are and knows how to get where you want to be. The key to learning the most from this experience is to ask questions that will elicit the best communication.

ARE YOU ROLE MODEL OR MENTOR MATERIAL?

The day I became a doctor, I began to carry myself in a different way. I conducted myself in a more proper manner and made better choices regarding my behavior. Because I work with children, I feel it is even more imperative for me to set a good example. But being a role model is not about what you do for a living, nor is it about trying to impress people. Being a role model is about living your life in a way that can be emulated by others. It is about deciding you want your life to have meaning, a purpose that is bigger than you. Do you use your talents and good fortune to improve the lives of others? Do you teach life lessons and instill values in those around you?

The people who benefit most from having a role model are those we love or encounter in our daily lives. We impart ideals and principles in our children, loved ones, and others we choose to share our lives with. This can involve being a teacher, volunteer, mentor, or just motivating people you meet on the streets. If you join an organization that has a mission to reach others, you can use your journey or story to inspire them on a larger platform.

Being the fabulous woman that you are, I am sure you have thought about how to use your life to better the lives of others. There are numerous ways to be a role model in your daily life or for a greater cause; the first step is for you to make that commitment. Role models and mentors are not perfect individuals. They are just imperfect people who have chosen to set a good example and educate others on the things they have learned and experienced over time, including their mistakes.

A number of women have asked me, "Who am I to be a role model? I am just a regular person!" I reply, "What is regular?" Regular to you may be amazing to someone else. You have a remarkable story that needs to be shared. The things you have accomplished may be the things that inspire someone to do better. Your everyday life can serve as motivation for someone who is looking for direction. And if you desire to become more influential and transcend what you consider a regular existence, then dare to start today. Look for opportunities to lend a helping hand or share your experiences with others.

All of the greats start out as regular people. Oprah Winfrey started out as an anchor on a local television station, but with hard work and tenacity, she became a billionaire who has helped millions of people around the world. Danica Patrick dropped out of high school and obtained her GED before becoming the most successful woman in stock car racing, inspiring women around the world to break barriers. But you don't have to be rich and famous to be an amazing role model. Even with all the people I have met in life, my mother is still my hero. It's not about fame or popularity when trying to make a difference in the lives of others. A true difference is made by taking an active interest in making someone's life better.

So what would make you a good mentor or role model? How can you inspire others? A genuine role model is one who has positive qualities and uses them to motivate others. Role models are leaders and encourage others to make changes for personal growth. You may not recognize the effect you have on others, the way you make the people around you better. You just trek along being fabulous, doing what you think is right; but you are an inspiration to many. Just being yourself can impact others as you naturally embody the traits of a role model.

Embracing these traits and living by these principles are a sure sign that you are a great mentor or role model:

1. Altruism

A good role model is concerned with the welfare of others. As an altruistic person, you are happy when you see others thrive and are disappointed when they suffer. Whether helping someone across the street, volunteering your time, or donating to a cause, being thoughtful and selfless in your interactions is an important part of being a role model. Helping others can be inconvenient at times, as you often have to use time and energy you would be spending on your own agenda. However, research shows that volunteering can actually improve our overall well-being, with less depression, pain, and chronic illness.[8] Altruism can also inspire others to make more of an impact.

You can play out selfless actions in your daily life or go above and beyond with an added commitment, but what truly matters is that you are able to put others' needs before your own.

2. Self-assurance

Accepting and loving yourself regardless of the path you have chosen is a part of growth and maturity. Taking pride in what you have accomplished builds confidence and further reinforces your belief in your ability to achieve further victories. Confidence is also an important aspect of being a leader. Believing in yourself without conceit inspires those around you to form their own goals. Your continued drive for success reinforces the idea that one person can succeed and make a difference.

3. Resilience

I am a true believer in "it is not about how you fall, but about how you rise." Having the courage to persist and continue to strive for success in the face of adversity is a sign of strong character. It is especially difficult to be resilient when your failures are witnessed or shared; however, being able to recover can motivate others to emulate you. You must recognize that things will not necessarily go as planned, so be flexible. Constantly reevaluate your path and goals to accommodate change. Hold on to your purpose no matter who or what tries to bring you down. Resilience is courageous and commendable.

4. Lifelong learner

Being an intellectual, a seeker of knowledge, is one of the things that sets role models apart. Role models are regularly in a position to instruct or lead, but to do that, they must have experience in the areas in which they are guiding others. Being an expert or pioneer in your field can inspire others to identify barriers that they can break down. Even when you are considered an authority, however, as a lifelong learner, you are never content with what you know. Reading for pleasure as well as to expand your knowledge and stay current is also important. Continuing to expand your area of expertise and broadening your horizons inspires others to get out of their comfort zone and challenge themselves to grow and progress.

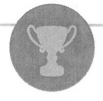

"Hold on to your purpose no matter who or what tries to bring you down."

5. Honesty

We've all heard the saying "honesty is the best policy." I think this means that when others look to you for direction, they want to know that you stand by your word. You believe in what you say and practice what you preach. One of the ways to make an impact in the life of another person is to be a consistent figure in their life and gain their trust. That occurs by following through and doing what you say you will do. How many leaders have fallen from grace because they were dishonest or hypocritical? We live in a forgiving society, but regaining trust and respect are very difficult. This also applies to mentors and role models.

6. Humility

Let's face it. No one is perfect. And nothing is more refreshing than someone you admire admitting to such. Showing your humanity by sharing your mistakes along with how you overcame them is often what others need to know to do better as well. When you think of great leaders, they are not the best at what they do but rather the most *appreciative*. Being humble and grateful when reaching your goals shows that you are worthy of being a role model. Don't get me wrong—it is great to excel at something, but it is even more admirable to have a humble attitude along with the talent. Being the best inspires individuals, but being exemplary with humility inspires the masses.

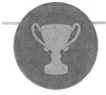

"**Being the best inspires individuals, but being exemplary with humility inspires the masses.**"

YOUR CHILD IS WATCHING

One area that lends to being a natural role model is already within the context of your home: being a mother. Being a mother provides the unique experience of having someone look up to you no matter what you have accomplished or experienced. Your relationship and interactions with your child shapes crucial fundamentals of his or her character, such as identity, self-esteem, and value system. Your child is watching and taking cues from you in order to learn about self and the world. By constantly observing you, your child learns how to behave and what behavior is appropriate and inappropriate. Ladies, let's be clear: you are your child's first role model, and the example you set can impact the type of person your child becomes.

I have talked to all types of mothers with different types of careers—engineers, artists, surgeons, and more. Most report that being a parent is more difficult than any other role they have ever taken on. The idea of another person's survival and outcome depending on the choices you make can be an overwhelming concept. Despite this challenge, many note that parenthood is the most rewarding thing they have ever done. A high percentage of the new patient consultations I perform as a child psychiatrist are with parents who need reassurance and education of what is expected, as well as direction on managing ordinary situations. However, every child is unique, hence every parenting experience being unique, too. No two paths are the same. You can read every book, manual, and blog out there for advice, but at the end of the day, you will face the daunting reality that you will not do everything perfectly. You will make mistakes, and your child will endure.

Being a good role model for your children is not about doing everything right. It is about setting the best example possible and using your mistakes as learning opportunities for everyone. You will forget to leave that dollar from the tooth fairy. You will slip and say a curse word, which your toddler will undoubtedly repeat at the wrong time. You will allow just a little more screen time when you have a lot to get done. But these momentary lapses will not tell the story. You will teach them right from wrong. You will treat people with respect. You will model appropriate communication of emotions. You will apologize when you have offended someone or hurt someone's feelings. You will keep trying even after you have failed. Imparting your fundamental beliefs and approaches to life will be the story. Your child will learn valuable lessons and become a functional person by seeing you in action, and that is what is important.

I am regularly asked how being a working mother impacts your child. This is an area that has been studied for years, and recent data has shown positive results. Children of career mothers show high academic achievement and benefits in conduct and social adjustment, and daughters possess a higher sense of competence. When fathers weigh in on the working-mother situation, they express that it leads to the children learning useful skills, improved quality of mother-child relationships, and benefits in the father-child relationships, as the fathers tend to pitch in more in childcare tasks.[9] The family as a whole seems to benefit from mom gaining satisfaction from career accomplishments. The working mother who ensures her children's needs are met while achieving life goals is a strong role model for her children.

Here are some of the other benefits of being a positive role model for your children:

Self-esteem

The formation of self-esteem is closely associated with parent figures. Your child is a blank slate when entering this world, so you are the guide in the development of self-esteem. When you respond to your children with loving words and actions as well as provide focused attention, you create a sense of value and significance. You are like a mirror reflecting your feeling of affection back to your child. When your child knows you care, it reinforces feelings of importance and a positive self-image.

Communication skills

"Use your words." That is a statement I commonly have parents articulate to their children. The more children are expected to use verbal communication, the more their communication skills develop. That's why it is so important for parents to be good role models in verbal communication. When you put your feelings and thoughts into words with your children, it demonstrates appropriate communication. Having regular discussions and encouraging your children to use their words from an early age gives them an opportunity to practice and cultivate the positive use of language. Children are like sponges—they pick up on the subtle nuances of language and behavior. If you repeatedly use inappropriate language or a negative tone in speaking with or in front of your children, they will learn to do the same. Be intentional in how you communicate with your child.

Emotional stability

One of the most difficult things about being a parent is knowing how to keep your cool with your children. You are almost out of the door on time . . . and there goes the pooping look. You are headed to the checkout line at the grocery store . . . and here comes the tantrum. Or your teenager is an hour late coming home again . . . but this time with a dent in the car. There are plenty of situations that will test your patience, and it is important that you use that patience. The way you handle difficult situations and deal with stress teaches your children how to manage their feelings. If you lose your temper or brood when you are upset, your children will likely exhibit similar behavior. Children will have tantrums and angry outbursts early in their lives while their emotional regulation is immature, but if you model appropriate management of difficult situations and teach them to control their tempers, they will learn how to use effective communication even during challenging situations.

Improved conduct

Many parents believe in the mantra "Do as I say, not as I do." They think that as long as they say the right things and tell their children the appropriate things to do, their kids will turn out fine. The reality is, children will mimic your behavior before they listen to your directions. Parents who exhibit negative behaviors, such as being disrespectful or talking down to others, are apt to have children who behave in a similar manner. Being able to effectively discipline your children and have them get along with others stems from you modeling respectful, well-mannered behavior, not just telling them what is right and wrong.

PAY IT FORWARD

One way to empower and inspire is to use the things you have learned to become a mentor yourself. Many successful individuals believe in the power of mentoring and paying it forward. Passing on knowledge and making a difference in someone's life is the ultimate sign that you have achieved success.

With our country shifting to a more selfish and ego-driven culture, we need more altruistic people who care about and invest in the lives of others. These thoughtful and selfless people will aid in building a more stable society in the future. You can be one of those people. You likely got to where you are today because someone took an interest or believed in you. It may have been your parents, a teacher, a coach, or a family friend. But some people don't have that someone and desperately need an extended hand. Some are struggling and trying to get up life's ladder with limited resources or support. Or worse, they may have no direction or goals at all.

Becoming a mentor can be extremely rewarding for you as well as for the person you take under your wing. Creating an atmosphere where you provide learning experiences for an individual is the key to developing a mentor-mentee relationship. These encounters provide the opportunity for your mentee to broaden horizons, gain skills, and change their outlook on life. Selecting a mentee who has an active interest in an area you embody or a skill you possess is crucial to being a relevant resource. That area of interest can be as simple as being educated or female or as specialized as being a scientist or an advocate for a specific interest group.

There are many ways to be an effective mentor on a daily basis. Showing a passion for the things that interest you can expose someone to something they have never experienced. You can try taking a coworker under your wing, signing up to be a professional mentor, or volunteering for an existing program. You may encounter mentoring experiences on your career path by working with interns. Use these everyday opportunities to pass on the knowledge you have gained in your life and to plant seeds in others.

You will notice that not only is your mentee progressing and learning new things, but you are also experiencing gains by sharpening your leadership and communication skills. Additionally, you will develop a sense of accomplishment and satisfaction in knowing that you are making a difference.

One mentor position that has been the most rewarding for me has been in working with youth in the juvenile justice system. Although my primary role is a psychiatrist, I have taken an active interest in certain youth who show promise and would benefit from having a mentor. I meet with them consistently and look for areas of opportunity to adjust their perspective or make positive changes. Some of the youth are just looking for someone to be genuine and empathic; they want an adult in their life to be present and listen.

In the mentoring capacity, I provide regular feedback and praise achievements (especially when made in overwhelmingly negative environments). When approaching them in a nonjudgmental manner, I am able to share my experiences and relay thought-provoking insights. Over time, I also have begun to make my own positive gains from the mentorship relationships. They have taught me to be thankful and appreciate the little things in life. My work with these youth has taught me more about resilience and courage than I could ever imagine.

Your evolution from an ambitious woman to Modern Trophy Wife and role model is an amazing journey. You will build relationships along the way that will aid in your development, but one of the most important relationships will be with your mentor. He or she will help you grow and reach your goals. As a result, the growth you experience, whether with your own children or in the community, will enable you to make a difference in the lives of others. There are many ways you can choose to foster another person's life and invest in them; just do it! You will enjoy it, and, like me, the life you end up changing may be your own!

THE MODERN TROPHY WIFE HALL OF FAME

There are a few women I admire and consider remarkable leaders and role models. They live their lives in an exemplary manner and emanate the attributes that a Modern Trophy Wife possesses. These brief profiles will give you an idea of what it takes to function as a positive role model in today's society.

1. **Melinda Gates:** Cofounder of the Bill & Melinda Gates Foundation, Melinda Gates has dedicated her life to being a champion for women. She is a leader in gender equality and invests in the future of girls around the world. As a wife and mother of three, she has redefined philanthropy by donating more than thirty billion dollars in grants since 2000. I applaud her commitment to her passion of advancing the lives of women and her perseverance in the field of global development.

2. **Michelle Obama:** Acting as the world's most famous wife and mother, Michelle Obama has used her position to advocate for a number of causes, including health and nutrition. While maintaining an aura of class, she has single-handedly challenged America's views of beauty, elegance, and strength. She is the epitome of a Modern Trophy Wife as she embodies confidence and seeks to enrich the world around her.

3. **Salma Hayek:** Known to some only as a beauty and actress, Salma Hayek has become a supporter and advocate for battered women's awareness. Mrs. Hayek earned my respect the day she breastfed a starving child in Sierra Leone in an effort to diminish the stigma of breastfeeding and bring awareness to the issue of world hunger. While some reacted in horror, I cemented a place in the Modern Trophy Wife Hall of Fame for her instead. She continues to work with and aid underprivileged children in Mexico.

4. **Sara Blakely:** I would be remiss to leave off the story of Sara Blakely. A wife and mother of four, Sara Blakely is now a billionaire in her own right. To my excitement, she took her $5,000 in savings and founded the Spanx shapewear brand, changing the lives of women around the world! She later created The Sara Blakely Foundation and is dedicated to the education of women in entrepreneurial training. She landed on my Hall of Fame because of her passion and tenacity. By believing in herself and not giving up, she turned an idea and $5,000 into a multimillion-dollar business.

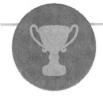

" **She is simply a dreamer who continues to learn and grow and uses her abilities to make the world a better place.**"

There is no blueprint for a Modern Trophy Wife. She comes in all walks of life. She is simply a dreamer who continues to learn and grow and uses her abilities to make the world a better place.

Notes

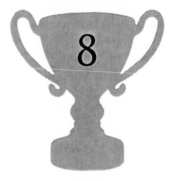

8

"You can't grow if you place yourself in a box."

FROM THE DESK OF
Dr. Metzger

THE MODERN TROPHY WIFE IS WILLING TO STEP OUT OF HER COMFORT ZONE

The greatness of a Modern Trophy Wife is achieved because she is constantly evolving to be her best self. This evolution happens when she gives a green light to new experiences. We have already covered when to politely say *no* earlier in the book, and now it's time to discuss when to respond with an enthusiastic *yes!* This means saying yes to new opportunities, new travels, new sports, new hobbies, new career moves, and new friends. All of these doors can lead to new adventures and advancements in your life. It's incredible what can unfold when you start taking footsteps outside of your comfort zone.

GO FOR THE "NEW"

Some of you may be rolling your eyes thinking this chapter doesn't pertain to you. You are saying in your head, "I'm not in my early twenties anymore. I'm past the stage of trying new things or making new friends. The college finding-myself phase of life has passed." That simply is not true. We are not too old to do something fresh and exciting. You have to

99

start moving in that direction to meet it. As you embrace new experiences, you will be pleasantly surprised by your talents and the unexpected joys.

I took a huge leap out my comfort zone (and my comfortable bed) when I decided to start exercising in the morning before work. I am talking early morning here—5:00 a.m. wake-up time. That sounds even earlier considering that more than four years ago, I was a night owl. I was up past midnight watching television or hanging out with friends on a weeknight! The only times I remember seeing the 5:00 a.m. hour was if I was on call at the hospital or had an early morning flight. Otherwise, I was deep in my dream stages during those hours. Then, I had children. My whole sleep-wake schedule got completely flipped. To all my mothers-to-be, this will likely happen to you; don't fight it. I have never treasured sleep more in my life, not even during my residency of taking thirty-hour hospital calls. I now find myself envying my boys as they get under the covers at 8 p.m.

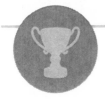 **" The greatness of a Modern Trophy Wife is achieved because she is constantly evolving to be her best self. "**

I had a dilemma, though. I realized that I wanted to get in shape but did not have the time to do it after work with the play-dinner-bath routine. It occurred to me (with the suggestion of my nutritionist and super-fit sister) that the best time to go to the gym is before the kids wake up. I started off really slow by going one or two times a week. I soon realized that I had more energy during the day. I also loved not having to think about going to the gym all day because it was already done. I didn't miss out on the evening routine with my kids, I got to exercise while they were still sleeping, and I had a mood-energy boost for the day. It was a win-win-win. I also became very fond of my new early bedtime after putting the boys to sleep. So far, this decision led to better health, better sleep, and just feeling better about myself overall. But that's not all I gained.

At the gym, I stepped out of my comfort zone and on to the treadmill. The treadmill and I have never been friends, actually closer to enemies if you measure the dread I had prior to getting on it. I also most definitely wouldn't have classified myself as a runner. I had participated in a 5K before as a brisk walk, but I never ran continuously. Now there I was, post two pregnancies and still struggling to drop those last ten to fifteen pounds. I realize the treadmill and I had to reunite to get rid of this baby weight. So I started running one or two days a week. I didn't love it, but it got easier.

One day, a gym buddy asked if I would like to do a 10K with her; I instantly said *yes!* It was a no-brainer. I didn't hesitate because it was a new experience that could bring positive benefits (health and mood). I'm also a sucker for trying things that people think I can't do. The jaw-dropping response of friends and family when I said I was running a 10K was worth it alone. I ran it slowly, and yes, I completed it. I loved the surge of accomplishment I felt after crossing the finish line.

The interesting thing I noticed about stepping out of my comfort zone is that once I started walking, I wanted to keep going farther. Since that race, I have run a 5K or 10K the first Saturday of each month. I now have five races under my belt, and I signed up to run a half marathon later this year. I am now the person asking for others to join me. I have reinvented myself. I became a race runner in 2016 and it began with one *yes!*

Do not be afraid of the new. The discoveries you may make about yourself and what makes you happy are worth giving it a try. This is the time. If you get an invite to do something you have never done, please don't be so quick to decline. A *yes!* may be life changing.

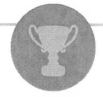 **"Do not be afraid of the new."**

VERTICAL CAREER MOVES

One major way to step out of your comfort zone is to consider a promotion, a new job, or even a new career. Have you ever heard that jobs are all based on who you know? That's not entirely true. Education and qualifications play a big role, but I do think having connections carries a lot of weight. People are more likely to root for someone they have met in person and liked. With this said, my next assignment for you is to start saying *yes!* to networking. I also want to dispel the myth that you need to be an expert saleswoman or social butterfly to network the right way. This is not true, either. Networking simply means introducing yourself and meeting other like-minded individuals.

A lot of people get so nervous about upcoming networking events. They fear what to say and just feel generally awkward about being in a room where they're expected to talk to people. This is usually why a small crowd can be spotted at the bar as people are trying to drink away their networking jitters. My advice is to take the pressure off. Be yourself. Rather than focusing on how you may appear to others, enjoy meeting new people and learning about them. The less self-conscious you are, the more approachable you will be and the more fun the event will be.

The reason I welcome networking events is because there is always a possible career opportunity that could come out of it. I'm not saying go to every networking event, but go to those that appeal to you. People of the same age group, same careers, or even similar backgrounds may be there. It's not a huge commitment. You can go and see if you like it. If you don't, you can always make an early exit. The possibilities in terms of career are worth the price of admission: saying *yes!*

 ## "Do not underestimate your value."

Career moves also require us to walk away from the familiar. Your mind can be your worst enemy when it comes to seeking jobs. You may see a job opening or a promotion and your first instinct is, "I'm not qualified enough for that," or "I probably won't get it anyway." When you think that way, you have already lost the job. There is no interview needed. Don't forget my tips about confidence! That is a key player to getting out of your comfort zone. You have to believe you're capable. You may be hesitant because it's a job in an arena you have never been in before. That makes it all the more exciting! Your faith cannot only lie within what you're currently doing; you must also have faith in what you are *capable* of doing. You won't know it until you try it.

I have worn the hat of executive coach for quite a few of my patients. I have learned that their own insecurities and self-imposed limitations are one of their biggest hurdles. Don't limit yourself. It is always good to be aware of new positions and new companies. There is nothing wrong with researching jobs in your field. You may be very happy with your current position and have been there for ten-plus years. That shows your loyalty, but do you feel it's the best that you can do? Would you be interested in more of a management role? Or do you prefer being out in the field working for a grassroots organization? Is there a nonprofit that you feel passionate about? A little inquiry never hurts.

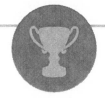

"Your happiness at work will transfer to happiness in your home."

Another important point is to know your value once an employer shows interest. Often, my patients are so excited to get an offer that they don't think to negotiate. You are a Modern Trophy Wife. Do not underestimate your value. The more you value yourself, the more they will realize what a prize as an employee you will be. I am speaking to those women within corporate America, but this also goes for my successful self-employed ladies. The services you provide are important and should not be valued any less because of your gender. (Okay, I'm stepping down from my girl power soapbox now.)

The basic point is that you should do something you enjoy. We spend approximately thirty-five percent of our waking hours at work, and this is only if we work a forty-hour week. That is more than a one-third of your life spent at the job. It should be doing something you like rather than just something you tolerate or do solely for the paycheck. If stepping out of your comfort zone professionally can mean a more fulfilling work life, don't just step—put on your sneakers and jump out of there! You may land in a job that is more rewarding. And your happiness at work will transfer to happiness in your home.

Travel, Meet, and Grow

I have found the most growth the further I am from my comfort zone. I have been blessed to excel in my career, but the most amazing thing has been my growth as a person. Meeting people, trying new things, and traveling to new places have all influenced who I am today. I have made friends in some of the most unlikely circumstances or chance meetings. I want you to remain open, too. I make a conscious effort not to choose my friends based on what they look like or how old they are. I have made friends with people who appear so different from me, yet we share so much in common, especially in how we cope and what we value. You can learn a great deal from such friendships. Stepping out of your comfort zone means embracing others who don't look like you, come from the same place, or view the world as you do. Open-mindedness and acceptance can expand your view of life and may even open more doors for you in the future.

The Modern Trophy Wife is also cultured. She has not only expanded her circle of friends and acquaintances but she has also widened the radius of her destinations. See new things. Go to places you have never been and experience a new culture. I have always thought that travel is one of the best ways to spend your hard-earned money. The experiences and memories made on these trips are priceless. When you look back on your life, I guarantee your travels with your family will be on the highlight reel. Gather your family and pull out a map. Choose somewhere you have never been.

My most memorable trip was to Australia in 2012. It was the best vacation, but not because of the food, the people, or the beaches. It was amazing because I was completely immersed in a new culture on the other side of the world. I learned how to throw boomerangs with Aboriginals, fed kangaroos, and watched the Australian Open under the Melbourne spotlights. It was mind-blowing because during the two weeks I was there, I was introduced to something brand-new every single day. The Australians greeted me with open arms and were just as curious about me as I was about them. They wanted to know about the States and asked questions about President Obama, and we chatted about their favorite American hip-hop artists. It was an exchange of laughter, knowledge, and most important, culture. It was a trip of a lifetime because it was something I had never done. Each day was a new adventure.

With that said, I urge you to start writing your own story and go somewhere you have only dreamed of. There will always be an excuse trying to stop you, like you're waiting until the kids get older or after you get a different job or after the ticket prices go down. Kick the excuses to the curb and just go for it.

The new experiences also can have a positive impact on your marriage. They bring spontaneity to the relationship to keep the spark going. They create new memories for you to share and get you out of a rut of always doing the routine. In couple's counseling, I usually have one person who complains of being bored with their spouse and feeling trapped in the ordinary. They talk about the old days when their spouse was willing to try something new.

My husband and I share that passion for the new, and I think that has kept our marriage healthy and entertaining. We are always on the search for a new restaurant and new travel spots, or even trying new sports. Planning new outings will give you both something to look forward to. It keeps the relationship fun but also builds creative ways that you can spend time with your husband. This is especially true when you have children, as it can be really easy to get caught in the web of the work-sleep-childcare routine. You have to live beyond that routine and literally fight your way out of the web. It takes an active effort not to become the boring and unhappy couple. Stepping out of your comfort zone with your husband helps to build a stronger relationship, and it's another way for you to enjoy each other's company.

You can start by looking in the local papers about events, see where the travel deals are, and chat with couples about their new ventures. You will discover not only ways to step out of your comfort zones but also fresh ways to enjoy your marriage.

OVERCOME THE FEAR

The main thing that makes people pause at the thought of stepping out of their comfort zone is anxiety. The anxious questions start popping into their head when faced with doing something new. *What if it doesn't work out? What if I can't do it? What if I fall on my face? What will people think?* Anxiety is a normal emotion when we do something we have never done. It's not realistic to expect that you won't be a little nervy about taking that first step. The important thing is to not let the anxiety overwhelm you to the point of stopping you in your tracks. Remind yourself that you can and will get through it. Learning how to overcome your fears makes more sense if you know the difference between good anxiety and bad anxiety.

Good anxiety is a natural human response. This response includes the surge of excitement, beads of sweat on our foreheads, heart racing, and chill we get down our spine before stepping on that stage, reading the first test question, meeting someone on a blind date, or taking a first stab at a new activity. This anxiety can also serve a protective role. It is what tells us to be cautious, and its biological name is known as the "fight or flight" response. Our natural "flight or fight" response is when our brain tells our body to go into defensive mode. It's what reminds us to avoid walking in dark stairwells, to stay away from suspicious people, and to look twice before crossing that busy intersection. Good anxiety is often a reflex and is actually beneficial. It keeps us aware and safe.

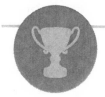

" Another person's failed attempt at a similar goal has no prediction on your results."

On the other hand, bad anxiety can do quite the opposite. It is limiting and often tries to derail progress. It's the "what if" fear that can prevent us from moving forward. The issue with the "what if" is it can scare us so much, but what we fear often never happens. That is why this anxiety is considered bad; it often gets people nervous for no reason. The fear is exaggerated compared to the chances of it happening in real life, as opposed to the fears of bad consequences that get people so worried it can literally be paralyzing. This fear stops them from ever stepping out of their comfort zone.

Bad anxiety can affect you mentally with the heavy worry but physically as well. It can affect the body from head to toe, causing headaches, muscle tightness, stomach cramps, chest tightness, and even tingling in the fingers and toes. Imagine trying to start a new venture with these physical symptoms taking over. This type of anxiety can make anything new almost impossible. The first step is to recognize it for what it is.

Bad anxiety is also very contagious. It is easy to take on the fears of others. People can talk you out of your dreams without you realizing it. Have you ever made a decision to move forward and then someone else's comments made you question yourself? This has happened to me in the past. I have been totally at peace with a decision and then someone's doubt soon creates fears that I never even thought of. I came to learn that their stories and doubts have nothing to do with me. I want you to apply this to yourself. Your talents are unique to you. Another person's failed attempt at a similar goal has no prediction on your results.

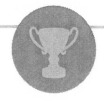

"Be careful with whom you share your destiny."

Ignoring discouraging remarks is necessary to not fall victim to bad anxiety. Giving in to the fears can pull you down to the point of eventually bringing you to a complete halt. You must disregard negative input. Discuss your dreams with only those you trust and who are positive. This is a hard rule for me. As I have mentioned, I am definitely a dream catcher, but I don't disclose my dreams to all who will listen. Be careful with whom you share your destiny. Some people, not having reached their own goals, may criticize your dreams. These Debbie Downers play no beneficial role in your journey. Tune them out and try your best not to get into your "dream mode" with them around.

I'll give you a personal example of how I made a conscious effort for my good anxiety to prevail over the bad. My first appearance on television was live. One summer Tuesday morning, I got the call from an HLN producer asking for my expertise on a family case. This was the acceleration I had wished for. But I was beyond anxious. Those thoughts of bad anxiety started knocking at my mind's door as soon as I hung up the phone. *What if I freeze? What if I say the wrong thing? What if I start to shake? What if I stutter? What if don't look at the right camera?* I literally was in my bathroom with the phone still in my right hand as all these thoughts raced through my mind at a full sprint.

So I spoke with a good friend and colleague about it. He said to me, "This is your moment. Save all that worrying for when you leave the studio." He was absolutely right. I immediately stopped the emotional spiral and reminded myself that this was a step toward my destiny. I realized that if I kept focusing on those bad "what if" thoughts, I would be doomed. This was live television, and there was no chance for do-overs. I wanted to make the best impression for the producers—not to mention the people watching across the world.

I decided to walk into the studio focused on this opportunity being a dream come true! I tucked those bad "what if" thoughts tightly away and got in front of the camera. The surge of excitement and nervousness was there, but it only motivated me to do my best. That was the good anxiety prevailing over the bad. The interesting thing is that the "what ifs" my friend told me to worry about later never happened. Unnecessary worry is the culprit that we must block to overcome our fears. And because I was determined not to let my worries get the best of me, I went on to make five appearances on HLN in that month!

I share my story to encourage you to tiptoe, step, or even jump out of that comfort zone. There is too much wonderful waiting outside of that fear. Start moving toward your destiny!

Notes

CHAPTER

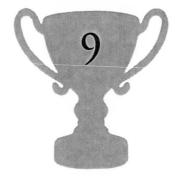

9

"Security within yourself is essential to healthy relationships with others."

FROM THE DESK OF
Dr. Gathing

THE MODERN TROPHY WIFE IS A SECURE WOMAN

The most valuable relationship you will ever have is the one you have with yourself. How you see yourself will grow and change over time, but learning to love and respect yourself for who you are is the ultimate goal. Accepting your identity, beliefs, and abilities is fundamental to your over-all functioning as an individual or as a healthy partner within a relation-ship. For any relationship to be successful, intimate or otherwise, it is es-sential that you are secure when entering into it. The idea many women have that someone will come into their life and make them feel complete is very romantic, but not at all sensible. Thinking that someone is going to round out your love for yourself, such as a husband, baby, or even a pet, is unrealistic. Building a life for yourself that brings you fulfillment and being able to share that with others is vital for contentment. At the end of the day, you are responsible for your own happiness.

That being said, everyone experiences bouts of insecurity at times. Am I making the right career move? How long will it take to snap back after giving birth? Should I be helping out more with my elderly par-ents? It is normal to have anxious thoughts at times, but confidence in your own competence gets you through these times. A secure woman understands that perfection is not the goal, and she does not compare herself to others. The only person you are competing with is the person you were yesterday.

Assessing your unique qualities is essential in evaluating your relationships. Do you feel complete as an individual separate from your relationships with others? Are you able to be vulnerable in relationships to improve communication and draw closer to one another? Does your behavior in your relationships reflect confidence and security within yourself?

Let's take a closer look.

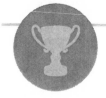

"At the end of the day, you are responsible for your own happiness."

INDEPENDENCE VS. INTERDEPENDENCE VS. CODEPENDENCE

I think it is great that women are embracing their independence. *Independence* is reveling in your individual characteristics, being free from constraints, and impacting your environment. Simply stated, independence is self-focused. It may manifest as celebrating educational attainments, enjoying financial freedom, and praising personal accomplishments. The process of becoming independent is healthy, as it allows you to discover your identity, build confidence, and determine your life path. The ability to listen to your own voice and applaud your accomplishments along the way is an important step to self-sufficiency. However, once self-sufficiency is attained and a relationship is sought, independence can impede the ability to connect with another person in an intimate way due to its self-focused nature.

Six Signs of Independence in a Relationship:

1. **You try to manage everything on your own.**
2. **You do not feel comfortable asking for emotional or financial support.**
3. **You have a hard time accepting your partner's opinions.**
4. **You do not like being held accountable to your partner.**

5. You do not incorporate your partner into all areas of your life.
6. You do not consider the dreams and goals of your partner.

Interdependence is the individual's ability to develop a relational view of themselves to others. It is when secure people form an attachment with one another and then divide the power equally within the relationship. Both parties are invested, make contributions, and are held accountable for their own actions. Interdependence is healthy in that the individuals involved are self-assured and do not depend on the other person to boost their self-esteem. It is easier to be vulnerable in an interdependent relationship as there is limited fear of someone taking advantage or attempting to gain emotional control.

There will be times when the needs of the relationship will take priority over the desires of self, but both people recognize that individual adjustments must occur to ensure the connection's success. However, it is important that personal goals and needs are supported in the relationship; each person must have mutual respect and appreciation of individuality. Interdependence requires looking at thought distortions, managing emotions, and adapting behavior as necessary for the good of the relationship.

Six Signs of an Interdependent Relationship:

1. You feel free to express yourself in the relationship.
2. You do not feel that you have to change your identity within the relationship.
3. You have a healthy balance of togetherness versus alone time.
4. You feel respected and supported in the relationship.
5. You are able to manage conflict in a healthy manner.
6. You are able to have your own dreams and goals in the relationship.

In contrast, *codependence* in relationships presents issues of control and balance. One partner may become accountable for the emotions and behavior of the other, and in turn, reciprocity does not exist. This creates an issue with vulnerability, as one partner cannot trust the other with their thoughts or feelings. A power struggle often develops, and opportunities for true connection and vulnerability do not occur. Independence is not supported, and individual needs are often not addressed because the relationship absorbs all of the focus and attention.

Communication is often hindered in an attempt to limit conflict, which further reinforces the pattern of each person's desires not being expressed or met. This dysfunctional way of relating to one another does not foster emotional or physical intimacy, and closeness suffers. Resentment, guilt, frustration, and hopelessness can build over time and further impact the connection.

Six Signs of a Codependent Relationship:

1. **You feel like you can't live without your mate.**
2. **You feel like your mate could not make it without you.**
3. **You feel your mate controls you.**
4. **You feel that you are constantly giving and not receiving.**
5. **Your happiness depends on the state of your relationship.**
6. **You feel you need the other person to take care of you.**

When examining your relationships, be sure to evaluate your role and what you are contributing. You are constantly teaching people how to treat you by the behaviors you tolerate from others. It takes two to form a pattern, so start by looking at your own emotional state and actions in relation to others. Even the most secure woman will have insecure moments, but exhibiting mature behavior is essential to maintaining functional relationships.

HEALTHY BOUNDARIES: READY, SET, MAINTAIN!

Security is the ability to feel safe or protected. Boundaries, spaces where you end and another begins, are how we create that sense of security. A boundary is a limit between you and another person. It is how you define what is acceptable and unacceptable in your life and relationships. Maintaining healthy boundaries in relationships is the key to protecting and taking good care of yourself while allowing the good things in and keeping the negative things out. Boundaries can be physical, such as your body, or mental, such as thoughts or beliefs.

This may be a complex concept for you as you may not have been taught how to set healthy boundaries. You may notice that you get caught up in the negativity of others or allow people to repeatedly take advantage of you. You may constantly feel violated or disrespected by someone, but you don't have the skills developed to set limits in order to maintain your own safety and security. On the other hand, some individuals create too many boundaries. They place emotional and physical guards in potentially healthy relationships, which keep good opportunities and great people at bay.

We learn what is appropriate and inappropriate from the people around us. In childhood, these figures are our parents. They are supposed to teach us right from wrong, what to accept and allow, and how to act within relationships. If you were not close to your parents, you likely had a parent figure and learned these lessons from him or her instead. If your parents or parent figures modeled improper boundaries, then chances are that you have some dysfunctional patterns within relationships. This can include emotional or physical abuse, allowing yourself to be controlled, being used or taken advantage of, or getting your needs ignored. These are all signs that you have not learned to set appropriate limits or to assert yourself with others. These poor boundaries often stem from having a poor sense of identity, no awareness of your own thoughts and feelings, or looking to others for approval.

Lack of assertion with others or emotional suppression can cause a buildup of negative feelings. Not expressing your opinion or avoiding conflict prevents resolution and finding peace, in your own mind and in your relationships with others. You end up absorbing the energy and problems of others, being taken advantage of, or giving up your needs entirely. Some of these situations may feel normal to you if you have been surrounded by dysfunction and participated in codependent relationships all of your life. You allow coworkers to push projects off on you, family to take money from you, or friends to constantly abuse your time. In intimate relationships, you allow your sexual boundaries to be crossed too soon, you are not treated with respect, or you are emotionally or physically abused. These indicate weak boundaries.

In contrast, if your parent figures were guarded or absent, you may be distrustful, have issues being vulnerable, or refuse to invest in others. These are signs that you may have too many limits with others or have rigid boundaries. Having rigid boundaries is like building a wall that others have to climb in order to get to the real you. With these inflexible boundaries, you refuse to let others in and convince yourself that you are content being alone or not dealing with others. Or you may have people in your life but do not let them get too close or see the real you in an effort to prevent getting hurt. Alienation of intimacy or not allowing others to get to know you can lead to disconnection or feelings of depression.

While you may convince yourself that you are fine with being alone because it does not require any work or emotional growth on your part, you will subconsciously yearn for companionship. Or perhaps you are married and aren't alone, but you hide your true feelings and keep things emotionally superficial. You exchange pleasantries or shallow conversation, but you are reluctant to provide any true expressions of emotion or sharing of feelings. This is a sign that your boundaries are too rigid and you are reluctant to build true intimacy.

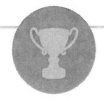

" As a Modern Trophy Wife, you must learn to maintain healthy boundaries while being vulnerable when appropriate."

As a Modern Trophy Wife, you must learn to maintain healthy boundaries while being vulnerable when appropriate. Learning to function and protect yourself within relationships is fundamental to maintaining confidence and empowering yourself and others. Perhaps you are currently working on setting limits or learning to open up. This guide will not replace therapy if you require further assistance in healing past wounds and trauma, but it can help you to assert yourself, demand respect, or feel more comfortable being vulnerable in your relationships.

Here are some basics to help you develop and maintain healthy boundaries:

116

1. **Identify unhealthy aspects of your relationships**

   There is no such thing as a perfect relationship, but there are healthy ones. Healthy relationships enhance or bring joy to our lives. Unhealthy relationships, or ones with unhealthy aspects, can cause discomfort or harm to those involved. You may feel uncomfortable with how being with someone makes you feel or with something you are asked to do. Or you may feel like you cannot be yourself, or that it is hard to let someone in. Unhealthy relationships can include someone attempting to control your behavior, making sexual innuendoes or gestures too soon, lack of commitment, asking to borrow money early in the relationship, or inappropriate displays of emotions, such as anger or irritability.

   Some behaviors or thoughts you may exhibit within a relationship are also inappropriate, such as feeling incomplete without the person, feeling uncomfortable expressing yourself, or being afraid to trust someone and let them in. In romantic relationships you may notice that you find fault with insignificant actions on his part and that he cannot live up to your expectations. Any signs that your relationships are unhealthy will cause you stress and likely affect other areas of your life.

   When you have created healthy boundaries, you are in a prime position to manage issues within relationships. Once you recognize specific patterns and behaviors, it is time to take action. Discuss these thoughts and feelings with the person in your life, and work on improving the negative aspects that you bring to the relationship.

2. **Detect boundary violations as they occur**

   Boundary violations occur when someone has tested the limits of your tolerance and with the potential to cause you harm. This is often not physical danger, although it most surely can be, but rather mental or emotional injury. The prelude to boundary violations can be boundary crossings. Boundary crossings are when people or situations challenge your limits or exhibit behavior that you feel is inappropriate. One example I hear about often is a husband repeatedly coming home later than the wife feels is appropriate for a married man. Her feelings toward this situation reveal a boundary she established prior to the relationship about what interactions after a certain time mean or what happens late at night. Because it is a preconceived notion, this belief may have nothing to do with the character of the person crossing the boundary, but it is now affecting your current relationship or situation.

Here is another example: your husband works in the sales and marketing industry, which requires after-hours' entertainment of new clients, but you do not take this information into account when his late nights make you feel uncomfortable. Boundary crossings are often simple to negotiate, but you do need to address them before you feel slighted or disrespected. Expressing your thoughts and feelings about a boundary and coming up with a solution that both parties can agree to often solves a boundary-crossing situation. If both parties are understanding, respectful, and willing to compromise, this can be a healthy experience for both people involved. These compromises can be especially helpful for someone with rigid boundaries who may need to learn how to be more flexible in relationships.

In contrast, a boundary violation, by definition, is harmful. It requires immediate attention in order to restore trust or safety. Violations can include someone sharing your personal information, constantly flirting despite your requests for it to end, or asking you to do something you are not comfortable with at work or within a relationship. Or violations may stem from someone being dishonest, unfaithful, or overtly threatening or abusive in your relationship. A foundation of security and trust is important in all relationships, so if those are compromised, then you need to address how to move forward.

3. **Develop a response to boundary violations**

Once you determine that your boundaries have been violated, you have to determine your response. The first step is to articulate the violation to the offender and communicate how it has affected you. This will ensure that there is no confusion about the action in question. During this acknowledgment process, you have to be clear about your feelings so that you don't get too caught up in the details or facts of what happened. Express your feelings of hurt, disappointment, anger, and frustration. I know communicating your emotions may be difficult, but it is necessary.

The next step is asserting a consequence for the action. This will depend on the level of the violation. For example, if your coworker continually pushes her work off on you and disrespects your time, an appropriate response may be to discuss this violation with her and alert her supervisor. Or if your male friend continues to make jokes and sexual innuendos toward you after telling him that it makes you feel uncomfortable, you might suggest to him that the two of you not hang out anymore until he can learn to respect your feelings.

Many individuals will not expect for you to acknowledge their boundary violations or for you to provide consequences, so expect a negative response initially. The offender may respond with hostility and play the victim, or he or she may avoid discussing the issue as they aren't used to being held accountable for their actions. No matter their reaction, make sure that you stick to your decision and uphold your assertions and consequences. Doing so will decrease the chances of similar behavior in the future. It may be awkward or even scary for you to discuss these situations, but it is necessary to ensure you receive the respect you deserve in your relationships. If the person responds appropriately and limits boundary violations moving forward, you can work toward regaining trust and security in that relationship.

4. Rid yourself of toxic roles and relationships

As a Modern Trophy Wife, you attempt to balance your roles. You have been in the moment, done some self-evaluation, and defined your own rules, but you still feel overwhelmed with your life or certain situations. You have lost your sense of self, or you no longer make your happiness a priority. You have set your limits and responded to boundary crossings when appropriate, but you continue to feel violated or disrespected. This may be a sign that you are still involved in unhealthy relationships or have people in your life who are continuously violating your boundaries.

It is necessary to evaluate your roles and the people in your life to determine whether the situation or relationships have run their course. Some people, opportunities, and roles come into your life for a season, perhaps to be used for further understanding of yourself and for your growth. But if you do not recognize that a relationship or situation is obstructive, you will remain stagnant.

One way to progress and seek contentment is to remove yourself from circumstances or people that have been hindering your growth and development. Perhaps your toxic work environment makes you come home from work daily feeling depressed and having low energy. Maybe someone in your life makes you feel worthless and unlovable, or you have been maintaining a friendship with someone who constantly takes but never gives. Some situations like these are immune to your attempts to provide structure and limits, or they are resistant to change despite your best efforts. This is when you must take action and move on.

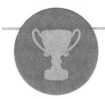 **"It is not uncommon for the most successful people to have stories of leaving situations, people, or careers behind in order to achieve greatness."**

It is not uncommon for the most successful people to have stories of leaving situations, people, or careers behind in order to achieve greatness. But many stay where they are and never reach their potential because they're afraid to leave circumstances or relationships behind. Fear of failure, fear of loneliness, or fear of not being good enough will prevent you from attaining the success you deserve. It is time to release your fears and free yourself from stagnancy. You are a Modern Trophy Wife primed to reach your life goals while you thrive at home, so step out of your fear, into security, and into your destiny.

Notes

CHAPTER

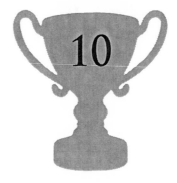

10

"A loving relationship is created by two people devoted to its success."

THE MODERN TROPHY WIFE IS EMPOWERED IN RELATIONSHIPS

Let's face it. Relationships are not easy. They take work, and I mean a lot of work, for them to have a chance at survival. There is a saying that relationships have to be 50/50, but I argue that it takes each person giving 100 percent for a marriage to thrive. This does not depend on how many other things you have going on, how you feel about your spouse that day, or how many children you have. Committing to your marriage as a priority is vital in its success. Nurturing your marriage like you do your career or your parenting is a daily process. It is important to develop your competence as a wife and invest in your marital relationship.

Many factors affect how you function within a marriage, including when you decided to get married, what you have observed of marriages prior to your union, and whom you choose as a companion. It is important to understand how these aspects influence your thoughts and behavior within the marriage. Once you recognize the impact these elements have, you can empower yourself to make informed decisions regarding the actions you take every day within your relationship.

Let's take a closer look at the factors that impact marriage.

> "There is a saying that relationships have to be 50/50, but I argue that it takes each person giving 100 percent for a marriage to thrive."

THE MARRIAGE SHIFT

With each passing generation, individuals are putting off marriage later or even entirely. Couples are now opting for alternative lifestyles, such as extended dating periods, long-distance relationships, and cohabitation. Surveys show that marriage is still a desired milestone for millennials at around seventy percent. However, that's much lower than their predecessors at ninety-one percent of baby boomers, eighty-seven percent of late bloomers, and eighty-two percent of generation Xers.[10] The rates have declined less dramatically for those with higher incomes and more education as this population continues to see the benefits of the institution, but even this group is choosing to marry later. Research shows the median age for first marriages is now twenty-seven for women and twenty-nine for men, up from twenty and twenty-three, respectively, in 1960.[11] This begs the question: what has changed?

Increased life choices

For years, couples married at young ages out of family or religious obligation. They had the support of their community but often little to show in personal gains. Women were uneducated, dependent, and with limited options in life.[12] Expanded liberties and opportunities for women, such as education and entering the workplace, were developed over time. With the resultant ability to take care of themselves, women were empowered to explore their options for personal and career satisfaction. Men also have become more focused on attaining life goals prior to tying the knot. These periods of independence have led to both sexes delaying marriage in an effort to experience self-discovery. It is now commonplace to desire fulfillment and experience more in life prior to settling down and focusing on personal ambitions.[13]

View of marriage material

As society progressed and the economy developed, more individuals began striving for the American dream: the big house, the white picket fence, the furry dog. To obtain these goals, people had to think more about development of wealth and income potential. It became obvious that marrying young and attempting to build a life while confronting the challenges of a relationship, career advancement, and child rearing were difficult. It is now considered undesirable to come empty-handed to the marriage table. Gone are the days when you start with nothing and create a life for yourselves. Whether it is education, maturity, skills, or means, it is now expected that you bring a strength to a relationship.[14]

Studies find that women with college degrees who waited until age thirty to get married earn significantly more than college-educated women who marry at younger ages.[15] The basis is likely an ability to focus more on self-care and life goals when single versus balance of ambitions when married. Women are now seeking to establish a career track prior to marriage so they can maximize long-term growth opportunities. Once in a wife and parent role, women may need to make certain sacrifices in their careers or life goals.

Women are also expecting men to be more financially and emotionally stable when entering into a serious relationship. The ability of a man to commit and have a mature mindset regarding the future are more important than ever when deciding whether he is the one. A secure job and career path are also key in viewing your partner as marriage material. These all come into play in deciding when to settle down, adding to the shift in marriage occurring later.

Outlook on marriage

The institution of marriage remains the standard for most. The idea of connecting with someone on a deeper level, committing to them, and braving whatever life throws your way together remains a popular sentiment. However, doing your own thing with no additional responsibilities or accountability can be an attractive sentiment. Independence is especially appealing to those of us who were raised in an era when independence and divorce were finally being embraced. The divorce rate peaked in the late 1970s and early 1980s, when the concepts of "no fault" and "irreconcilable differences" became legal.[16] Before that time, a spouse had to prove adultery or cruelty in a marriage for divorce to be approved. Now, a person can leave a marriage due to not being content. Combined with additional rights granted to women, the ability to freely divorce became a symbol of legal and emotional freedom.[17]

Some of us, me included, experienced the effects of this type of thinking. Growing up with divorced parents alters your view of marriage. Marriage was once seen as a fairy tale of sorts, being saved from a life of loneliness with love and a promise of forever. But when witnessing that love turn into loathing, disgust, or detachment, you start to consider the realities of the institution. You start to consider the effects of things such as finances, distance, and personalities on the story. Marriage starts to look less romantic and enchanting and starts to look more challenging and possibly impractical. Fear and anxiety surrounding this level of commitment can develop, leading to more cautious and pragmatic behavior.

But when the chips are down and the idea of life in older age approaches, many start to change their tune. The comfort of not having to face adversity or be vulnerable starts to give way to a longing for companionship. A secure woman recognizes her desire for commitment, but she is able to manage her expectations. She knows that life is not make-believe, but she is able to create her own little love story. And so while at a lower rate and occurring later than our predecessors, the marriage force continues!

THE EFFECTS ON RELATIONSHIPS OF MARRYING LATER

Seeking the ideal mate

I have encountered many women who have expressed this concept of waiting to marry in order to find her ideal mate. Some have a type of man in mind that they thought through on many occasions, others with an actual checklist they have written down. The idea is similar in that these women refuse to settle for just any ol' guy. In recent studies, the quality that women rate most desirable in a man is a secure job at or above her level, followed by similar ideas in raising kids.[18] This lends itself to the idea that we may be moving toward a society that practices assortative mating.

Assortative mating is the tendency of like people to mate with one another, or that people marry people like themselves in order to mate. This tends to bring together people with comparable education, earning potential, values, and lifestyle. You are choosing to be with someone with similar passions, interests, and life goals. It is now more common to look to a marriage with a person you enjoy spending time with and for companionship. To capture a person with these qualities and values, women are marrying later to know their partner's capabilities and vision.

Gender role evolution

If the statistics continue in the current trend, half of American households may have a woman as the principle wage earner by 2025. Women are earning college and postgraduate degrees at higher rates than men, leading to a closure in the wage gap. Nowadays, marriage occurs with men and women who have been in the workplace and living independently longer, so they both should be more capable of performing domestic tasks. Despite women's high educational attainment and men's increased proficiency in self-care, household duties are primarily considered a female responsibility. Even wives who earn more do significantly more housework and childcare than their husbands.[19]

Of late, there have been some dynamic shifts in views regarding gender roles. Men are now aspiring to be more hands-on fathers in addition to being breadwinners, and women are more open to being primary breadwinners. Gender roles and threats to identity have become one of the leading causes of conflict within modern marriages. A mate who aligns with your interests and provides companionship does not mean you align in gender role ideals. Couples can lack communication regarding philosophies on important matters that build the foundation of relationships. Working couples regularly struggle regarding division of household labor, childcare, and financial distribution. These discrepant paradigms in gender responsibilities can present discord in relationships if left unresolved.

The key to resolving gender role conflicts is examining your beliefs and looking for a compromise. For example:

Scenario 1

Problem: Jane is a hard-working female executive, wife to John, and mother of two. She often works long hours, volunteers at the local shelter, and has multiple hobbies that she enjoys participating in with her friend network. John is a writer with flexible hours who enjoys being in the home. He feels that women should manage all domestic tasks, such as cooking, cleaning the home, and getting the children to activities. Jane knows that John expects her to manage the household, so since her role was expanded at work, she stays up late to finish projects, has been volunteering less at the shelter, and has not spent any time with her friends. John has been frustrated lately as he and Jane have not been sexually intimate in months.

Solution: John does not understand that Jane's libido is directly linked to her energy level. Jane has been overworked since her position expanded, and she continues completing her same tasks at home. This increase in her demands have led to mental and physical exhaustion, a common deterrent to female sexual desire. Jane needs to vocalize that although she does not mind being the primary caretaker and household manager, she needs some backup with her heavier load at work. It may not be obvious to John that her increased work load has thrown off her balance, and that he may need to step up in some areas to provide her some relief. Ideally, they need to talk about her limits to determine compromises that work for both of them so that Jane can give more to their emotional and physical intimacy. John's primary complaint was a lack of intimacy, so Jane should frame the conversation around how his helping in the home can provide more opportunities for self-care, which could result in more energy to give to the sexual relationship.

Scenario 2

Problem: Mary is a business analyst, wife to Michael, and mother of one. Michael was laid off from his high-paying marketing position nine months ago. They are doing fine financially as they had both put money away for emergencies, but they have had to cut back on lavish spending. Michael has been at home while looking for work and has been excited about pitching in more with the household duties and childcare. Mary has appreciated the help with the domestic duties, but she has been irritable and cold to Michael for the last few months. She has noticed that her attitude surfaces whenever Michael gives directives for how she needs to spend money. She admits his guidance has been frustrating, although he usually made these financial decisions in the past.

Solution: With Michael's recent layoff, Mary is now the primary breadwinner in the home. This conversion, however, has not come with any identified shifts in his role. Michael has continued to make the financial decisions and has even picked up some slack in the household duties. Mary is clearly experiencing issues with her respect level for Michael now that there has been a swing in the balance of financial power. She admires that he has undertaken domestic tasks, but it has not helped her struggle with no longer viewing him as the "man of the house." It takes a very secure woman to manage this sort of dramatic transformation in dynamics. If previously financially dependable, you relate to your significant other as someone who can provide security. Changes in this ability may lead you to feel resentful, oppositional, and possibly angry with the unexpected alteration to the stable life that the two of you built.

Mary and Michael have lacked communication of the important ideals being tested. Mary's frustration with the evolution of her role and the impact to her security needs to be discussed. Simply acknowledging her feelings may provide some relief, but she also needs to talk about how to restore her feelings of safety. Should she be able to have more financial decision making during this time? Should they be more collaborative in how the childcare duties are divvied? Each couple's compromises to restore relational balance will be unique, but the key is to be honest and open about your feelings and needs.

Scenario 3

Problem: Susan is a teacher who met the love of her life, Steven, a school superintendent, at a conference. They share many interests; aside from their passion for educating children, they are both nature enthusiasts and animal lovers. Susan is pregnant with the couple's first son, and they are very excited. One day, Susan provides Steven with various options to review for their child to attend day care. At that time, Steven shares that he wants her to stay at home with the child for the first year of his life. Susan is shocked and angered by this suggestion as she was set to be promoted to department head shortly after returning to work. She has never considered the possibility of being a stay-at-home mother and wouldn't even know how to make that work. Since that conversation, Susan and Steven have frequently argued over who is going to do the dishes or other household tasks, and they have been eating out as no one has prepared dinner.

Solution: Susan and Steven are a common example of a couple who has married without discussing their values on gender roles. The couple shares common interests and passions, but they did not explore their thoughts on the fundamental view of how men and women function within a relationship. Many couples marry for companionship or because someone makes them happy without examining basic compatibilities. When confronted with an issue that challenges their essential beliefs, couples are tested in their ability to be flexible. Although you may respect your partner's views on gender roles, you may not want to conform to their ideals. A secure individual is able to accommodate some of her partner's values in her decision making, but it is difficult when the couple is not having conversations that promote this sort of understanding.

Susan and Steven need to discuss their opinions surrounding gender roles and expectations. It may be that once Steven talks about why he feels it is important for a mother to be at home with her child for the first year of life, she may totally agree and be open to it. Or if Susan describes her career path and ambitions to Steven and how she feels that she can balance that with successful parenting, he may be sold.

Some scenarios could provide a compromise, such as staying home for a little longer than planned but not quite the full first year. While having these conversations, Susan and Steven need to elaborate to include their ideas of who should be doing what in regard to domestic tasks. When conflict was presented in their relationship, everyone abandoned the household ship! That is a clear sign that there was no stated or implicit accountability for those tasks.

As you can see, communication and understanding is at the center of each of these solutions. When in a relationship, it is important to verbalize your feelings and thoughts in a respectful manner so that a resolution can be determined. Suppressing your emotions and desires leads to inappropriate behavior and poor problem solving. Conflicts are unavoidable, but communication is the tool you use to navigate these difficult situations.

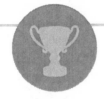

" **Conflicts are unavoidable, but communication is the tool you use to navigate these difficult situations.**"

FERTILITY MATTERS

One area that has allowed for the possibility of marrying later is the progression of technology. Technology impacts the way we communicate, how we view ourselves, and our perspective of the world. Gone are the days when everyone was born and raised in the same town or everyone lives right down the street from their loved ones. Now it is common to move about, travel the world, and seek new opportunities.

The age of information exchange has also broadened our horizons and allowed a new era in the way we define and create our family. More couples than ever before are waiting until later in life for childbirth and child rearing.[20] This stems from advances in technologies allowing conception in later years, such as in vitro fertilization, oocyte cryopreservation (egg freezing), and egg donation. It is also more socially acceptable to have children through adoption and surrogacy, some even facilitated or sponsored by the workplace. These advances have allowed more flexibility in creating and building a family, especially in later-life couples.

As many desire to conceive in the traditional manner, marrying and procreating later have led to a surge in couples dealing with infertility. According to the U.S. Department of Health and Human Services, approximately ten to fifteen percent of couples in the United States are infertile.[21] Infertile couples are defined as not having conceived after at least one year of regular, unprotected sex. Studies show that a woman's fertility starts to drop after she is about thirty-two years old, particularly after age thirty-five. Male fertility progressively drops after age forty. So despite couples feeling less pressured to marry, they do, however, continue to feel the pressure to conceive. For the ones who do not give in to the pressure of the ticking biological clock, they may later encounter issues when ready to bear children. Even the most secure woman can be devastated when faced with the reality of infertility.

But here are some reasons you should not fret!

1. **Infertility may be reversible**

   Many causes of female infertility are things that are reversible. Excessive exercise or weight abnormalities, certain medications, medical conditions, and uterine growths are related to infertility and can be corrected with assistance. There are also hormonal and reproductive track abnormalities that can be addressed with medical intervention.

2. **He can take action**

   Studies show that at least one-third of infertility cases are related to male causes.[22] These can be anything from sperm production or functional issues, lifestyle issues (for example, smoking, excessive alcohol use, marijuana, or steroids), or illness. Urge your guy to also get evaluated for ways he can improve his fertility.

3. **It's better to have fun trying**

   Many couples report that the stress of procreating alone stood in their way of conceiving. Sex can start to become routine, unromantic, and mechanical when in the process. The repeated negative pregnancy tests can become demoralizing. The stress of the situation itself, compounded by normal life stressors, can lead to further issues with fertility. Stress reduction techniques and lifestyle changes often allow couples to conceive who couldn't before. Lowering stress to increase fertility can be as simple as a massage, acupuncture, or weekend getaways.

4. **There are other reasonable options**

I know, I know. You want to conceive your child the good old-fashioned way. But when it comes down to it, there have been dramatic developments in assisted reproductive technology. Contact your gynecologist for an evaluation to discuss your options.

Let's Talk About Sex

It is impossible to discuss relationships without broaching the subject of sex. Physical intimacy is one of the most important indicators of how an intimate relationship is functioning, but for some reason, it has almost become a taboo subject! How often a couple engages in regular sexual activity can suggest the health of the connection.[23] This doesn't mean comparing yourself with newlyweds who just returned from their honeymoon. But in relation to when you were the most secure and happy, how often you are having sex at any given point can be a barometer of your relationship well-being. Whether once a day, once a month, or once a year at baseline, it is important for both individuals to feel that their needs are being addressed.

Some individuals feel that other forms of physical interactions are just as or more important than sex, such as kisses, massages, or playful wrestling. Similar to emotional needs and security, both individuals should have sexual desires they feel comfortable communicating. If partners do not feel that their physical needs are being addressed, then they may shut down emotionally. But addressing sexual desires does not mean having sex whenever you see fit! It means having an honest and open dialogue about your requests and wants, and seeing where to compromise to suit both parties.

Here are just a few of the suggested benefits a healthy sexual relationship:

Better mood

It is no surprise that sex makes you feel good. But there is not just a physical reason for that; there's also a chemical one. During sex, the body releases dopamine, a neurotransmitter involved in the reward system. The reward system is involved in everything you do that brings you pleasure and positivity. In addition to dopamine, the body also releases oxytocin during sex. Oxytocin is involved in attachment and bonding, and it aids in feeling good during and for some time after sex. Sounds like a great reason to cuddle up in the bedroom!

Better sleep

If you orgasm, the hormone prolactin is released. Prolactin has many effects on the body, but one in particular is sleep induction. Prolactin levels are the highest during sleep, and studies show that prolactin level peaking after orgasm leads to feelings of tiredness.[24] Add that to the list of reasons to keep going until you experience the big O!

Reduced stress and anxiety

One of the best reasons to participate in sexual activity is due to its stress-relieving properties. Positive physical contact with your mate has been shown to lower hormones associated with stress and to reduce symptoms of anxiety. Studies show that people who have had sex recently are better able to handle stressful situations.[25] And it isn't just the actual deed that counts, as other forms of physical intimacy with a partner, such as hugging, kissing, and massages, also have been shown to reduce stress. Nurturing the intimacy in your relationship can decrease anxiety overall, so go ahead and get a little closer.

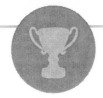

" **Nurturing the intimacy in your relationship can decrease anxiety overall, so go ahead and get a little closer.**"

In my experience, even with open dialogue regarding physical intimacy, couples regularly place their sexual relationship on the back burner. Instead, they often focus on things they consider more immediate or urgent, such as work, children, or passion projects. During these times, physical chemistry is not always present as there are other things on your mind. You are not mentally in tune. Studies show that there are more sexless couples walking around than you would guess, ones that have sex less than ten times per year![26]

" **What is most important is that both individuals are in tune and on the same page regarding where you are sexually."**

Of course, one number doesn't define a healthy sex life. A healthy sex life is variable and depends on each couple's ideals, desires, and beliefs regarding sex. Also to be taken into consideration are age, life circumstances, and personal preferences as sex drive waxes and wanes across the life span. What is most important is that both individuals are in tune and on the same page regarding where you are sexually. It can be scary or frustrating if things are not where you feel they should be, even though it is not one person's fault. If one or both partners do not feel comfortable with where the sexual relationship is, it can be difficult to get things back on track.

Here are some ideas to get you started and back into the bedroom:

1. **Keep an open mind**

   All of us have our preferences and things that we like to do. But over time, that can lead to staleness or boredom. Whether trying new positions, trying a new time of the day, or changing your setting, be open to trying something new or different. Changing things up can keep things spicy and reenergize your sex life.

2. **Trade places**

   If one person is usually the initiator, switch things up. Having the other person get things started can boost the chemistry of the encounter. Maintaining a sexual relationship takes effort from both parties, so having the individual who rarely initiates take initiative can reinvigorate the spark.

3. **Nurture the emotional connection**

   With all of the things going on in your life, you may not be foster-
   ing the mental and emotional connection in your relationship. Try
   to remember what made you fall in love in the first place. The little things like spending time alone, laughing together, and having
   some fun can help to restore the chemistry. Rebuilding the foundation of the relationship makes you feel more secure and aids in
   conflict resolution. Resolving issues and regaining confidence will
   bring you closer, and you will be more apt to want to get back into
   the bedroom.

4. **Put it on the calendar**

   I know, I know. Scheduling sex seems to take all the fun out of it.
   It seems unnatural and rigid. But couples who have a regular time
   set aside are more likely to have sex than those who just go with
   the flow. Having a sex date does not limit you from having sex at
   other times, but it does ensure that you carve out moments to spend
   together for closeness and intimacy. So pull out those planners and
   get to scheduling!

5. **Check in**

   Regularly checking in with your partner on how you feel about the
   relationship as a whole, including the sexual aspect, promotes increased communication and engagement. Many couples assume
   that they know what the other person is thinking or feeling, but over
   time, we may be less able to read our partner, or there may have been
   shifts in thinking. This is the perfect time to discuss new things that
   you may want to try, or bring back an old trick you've been missing!
   You may also use this time to confront any unmet needs in the relationship in general.

These are by no means all the factors that go into creating a successful relationship. They are just some of the areas that impact the relationship of a Modern Trophy Wife. You will have ups and downs, good
days and bad, accomplishments and challenges. It is important to remain
encouraged. No matter what path you have chosen or where you are in
your journey, using these tools to prioritize the health and communication in your marriage will help you withstand the test of time.

Notes

Conclusion

The Modern Trophy Wife is not a style or a profession. It is a state of mind. It is the woman who is juggling, but doing it with grace. The Modern Trophy Wife is a champion.

The drive for writing this book was for you to not only gain tips to improve your lifestyle but also to learn how to realize how amazing you are. Our balancing act of marriage, career, fitness, self-care, and for some motherhood is no easy feat. You are a star for being able to perform in all of these roles. The goal of this book is to teach you how to shine the brightest. Your light will not only shine in your marriage but also with your family, friends, and colleagues. You set an example for women who yearn to have it all.

The Modern Trophy Wife dispels the myth of the impossible balance of career, family, and self-care. The Modern Trophy Wife is the mom at the PTA meeting, the wife out on date night with her husband, and the supervisor killing the presentation in the boardroom. She is very much real and inspiring to others who wish to be in her shoes. And these shoes are not just the high heels of a traditional trophy wife. The Modern Trophy Wife's shoes are sneakers, hiking boots, comfy flats, dancing shoes, and many more. Her footsteps make a lasting imprint wherever she goes.

The key is that the Modern Trophy Wife preserves her joy. The reason she sparkles is not because of all she can do, but how she does it. Her humility and strength are immediately evident. She prioritizes her self-care, support network, and the union of her marriage. She has the perseverance to work toward life goals and the fearlessness to step out of her comfort zone. The ability to do this while wearing so many hats is possible, and the confidence she displays in these roles is what earns her the trophy—not just her beauty.

We have explored the redefinition of the trophy wife in modern times. She is not just arm candy for her husband but rather stands alongside him with their arms interlocked as a power couple. Her success is not defined as just being a Mrs. but by oh so much more. "Smart is the new sexy"—and the educated and empowered woman is now the sought-after bride.

The tips in this book are to highlight and strengthen the attributes you already possess. The Modern Trophy Wife is a role model yet humble, strong yet vulnerable, a leader and a friend. She is *you*.

Notes

BONUS CHAPTER

"Trophy status is not about getting the ring; it is about embracing your journey as a vibrant woman."

THE MODERN TROPHY WIFE STARTED AS A TROPHY WOMAN

A Modern Trophy Wife is not about looks or size. And it is definitely not about you or your significant other's bank account. A Modern Trophy Wife is an attitude, a way of life, and a goal to be a better person tomorrow than you are today. This process does not begin on your wedding day or the day you become a mother. All Modern Trophy Wives were once trophy women. A trophy woman embodies many of the qualities discussed in this book, but she has not yet stepped into the wife or mother role. She is confident, demands respect, and balances living in the moment versus preparing for the future.

While writing this book, we were given feedback from unmarried ladies who felt they embodied the traits of a Modern Trophy Wife. You may be one of those women. You are mastering self-care, working to establish yourself as an amazing force, and living as a role model for others. You travel to destinations near and far, experience new things, and are learning to create balance. You are out there discovering your identity, fulfilling your purpose, and striving to reach your goals. You aspire to be great, to do more and be better. You may be focused on finding the person to spend the rest of your life with, or you may not be particularly interested in being a wife or mother at this point.

Whether you aspire to marry now or are concentrating on building your own foundation, there are many aspects of living like a trophy woman. Everyone's path and journey will look different, but we are here to help you get started on the path of living like a trophy woman.

ENJOY YOUR SINGLE EXPERIENCE

When I was a child, my mother used to say, "Do not rush to be an adult; enjoy being a kid." I didn't know what that meant at the time, but I eventually came to understand the meaning of her statement. Being an adult is amazing as it comes with freedoms and experiences that you are not able to do as a child, but it also comes with numerous responsibilities and obligations. You have to take care of yourself. You have to worry about your future. You have to protect yourself. As a child, you don't see those things; you see the glamorous aspects of being an adult. You can come home when you decide. You can hang out with whomever you want. You can spend your money on what you choose. The grass looks greener on the other side, and this is also true for singles.

Single women often idealize marriage and motherhood. You see the glamorous aspects of marriage, such as having a companion, adorable children, and building wealth. You feel like no matter what you achieve, none of it matters until you can add the accomplishment of being a wife and mother. It is engrained in women to think of life goals as what we do until we reach the ultimate goal of marriage. And this belief is regularly reinforced by those around you. You call your family to tell them about your promotion, and they ask whether you have been on any successful dates lately. You tell your coworkers about the wonderful trip you are planning, and they ask whether will be bringing a companion. Your friends ask what you will be getting for Christmas, followed shortly by "it better finally be a ring."

But what these same people do not tell you is that they often envy your life. They are jealous of your ability to focus on your own needs and not answering to anyone. They don't discuss the realities that come with having a family, such as being accountable to another person, managing relational issues, and the compromises made for the good of the family unit. As mentioned throughout this book, marriage and motherhood are wonderful experiences, but they come with additional responsibilities.

A trophy woman embraces her single experience. Stop wishing for a life that you do not have, and enjoy the one you do have. Be content with your journey, as you will live it only once.

There are many advantages to being single that you may not have thought about. Here are a few:

1. **Choosing how to spend your time**

   There is nothing more freeing than being able to choose exactly how to spend your time. When you are single, you get to organize your schedule exactly the way you want. You can work out in the mornings or late at night, you can hang out with your friends in the middle of the week, and you can stay late at work as often as you need to. Being able to spend your time how you prefer is an advantage single women often take for granted.

2. **Spending your money the way you see fit**

   This one is a very important concept. When you are married, "your" money becomes "our" money, and it must be managed as a team. When you are single, you can squander or splurge at your will. Often, there are fewer things you are financially responsible for and fewer people to have opinions regarding where your money should be directed.

3. **Managing your household the way you like**

   Do you like doing all your cleaning on the weekends or laundry once a week? No problem! Everything will be right where you put it and not bothering anyone else. You can get to it when you can or organize a cleaning schedule. Either way, it's on your own terms and your own mess to deal with.

4. **Being as social or solitary as you want**

   Whether you feel like hanging out or want to Netflix and chill, it is up to you. There are times when you feel like being out and about or other times when you want to curl up with a good book by yourself.

You do not have to attend social events out of obligation, or stay home with a partner when you feel like partying. It's up to you!

5. **Prioritizing what is most important to you**
   While single, you are able to decide what you are most passionate about and focus on those things. You may decide to place more attention on your spiritual development, focus on career advancement, or be more health conscious.. You do not have to worry about getting someone else on board or competing with your priorities.

6. **Being spontaneous**
   Your coworkers decide to head out after work for happy hour. No problem. Your girlfriend invites you on an all-expenses-paid trip for the weekend. Awesome! Your sister decides she wants to come over tonight. Yay! You can make last-minute decisions whenever you want as you only have your needs to consider. You do not have to plan for a sitter, discuss it with the hubby, or catch up on DVR because you are good to go.

7. **Sleeping when you want, and often!**
   This one is a no-brainer. It is obvious that with a husband or child, you may have to alter your sleep patterns or stick with a more convenient schedule. With all of the responsibilities, you also may not have as much time to devote to sleeping. So go ahead and get your zzz's now!

This is not an exhaustive list by any means. It is just a few examples of the things that are great about the single experience. In the spirit of my mother's advice: "Do not rush to be married with children; enjoy being single."

DATING WITH DEAL-BREAKERS

Most women have done it. And I am no different. Many of us have come up with a checklist of the qualities our ideal man possesses, the list of things we are looking for in our future mate. Some of you have written this checklist out and added to it over time. Others have it mentally engrained and memorized. You use this list to evaluate each man you meet, sizing him up in just minutes. One checkbox off, and he is discarded. Or you may use it to justify a case for not even giving someone a chance at all.

Here was mine:

1. Tall (preferably over six foot two)
2. Christian
3. Athletic with a good body
4. Good looking
5. Values family
6. Educated
7. A good person
8. Great job
9. Loves to travel
10. Loves sports
11. Loves the movies
12. Has a sense of humor
13. Fun!!!
14. Has his own place
15. Honest
16. Between the ages of twenty-eight and thirty-eight (preferably between thirty and thirty-five)
17. Mature
18. Secure with himself (but not arrogant)
19. Willing to commit

If you have never made this kind of list, that is fine. You are actually one step ahead of what I am about to tell you to do. Ladies, I want you to take this list and throw it away. Yep. Rip up that paper. Delete it from your phone notes. Erase it from your memory. *Why would I do that?* you ask. Because this list is holding you back. It is a romanticized ideal of the perfect man for you. Or even worse, it is based on a real man you dated or encountered who did not work out, and now you are mentally attempting to replace him. If there is one thing you should learn from reading this book, it is that no one is perfect. No situation is perfect. So the idea that we can come up with a list of superlatives and expect that to translate into the exact person we are meant to be with is impractical.

But there *is* a list you need to make. You need to write this one down, take a mental picture, and commit it to memory. This is your list of deal-breakers. Your absolute have-to-haves and things you cannot accept. It should comprise of principles and qualities you refuse to negotiate. This is not the place you put the things you prefer or things you can compromise. This list should be much shorter than your original checklist. That one included your desires and wishes versus your musts. When creating this list, make sure whatever you include is measurable. It was great that I wanted "a good person," but that is very subjective. Does that mean that he volunteers on the weekends or adopts animals from the shelter? No clue! It was just something I felt I would know when I saw it. And that may have been true. But this list is for things you are able to readily identify when you interact with a person.

Here was my list of deal-breakers:

1. **Christian and attends church regularly**
2. **Enjoys spending time with family**
3. **Treats me with respect**
4. **Makes me laugh**
5. **Is willing to commit**
6. **Is not dishonest**
7. **Is not arrogant**

As you can see, this list is cut down to must-haves. This list is not your be-all and end-all; it is the foundation on which you decide whether someone is relationship material. It helps you to evaluate whether someone is worth spending your valuable time with. Living like a trophy woman means not wasting your time on people or situations that are not worthy of your attention.

If you like some of the concepts we've addressed here, pick up a copy of our second book in the Modern Trophy Life Series, *Dating Like a Champion* (Spring 2017), in which we explore how to balance living in the moment while preparing for the future in your dating life.

Notes

Endnotes

1. Meilena Hauslendale, *Stop Complaining: Guide to Living Life Instead of Complaining About It* (Raleigh, NC: Lulu Press, Inc., 2009).
2. Andrew Perrin, "Social Media Usage: 2005-2015," Pew Research Center, October 8, 2015.
3. David D. Burns, *The Feeling Good Handbook* (New York: Plume, 1999).
4. F. Ozbay, D. C. Johnson, E. Dimoulas, C. A. Morgan, D. Charney, and S. Southwick, "Social Support and Resilience to Stress: From Neurobiology to Clinical Practice," *Psychiatry (Edgmont)* 4, no. 5 (2007), 35–40.
5. Ibid.
6. Katerina Johnson and Robin Dunbar, "Pain tolerance predicts human social network size," *Scientific Reports* 6, Article 25267 (2016).
7. B. N. Uchino, M. Carlisle, W. Birmingham, and A. A. Vaughn, "Social Support and the Reactivity Hypothesis: Conceptual Issues in Examining the Efficacy of Received Support During Acute Psychological Stress," *Biological Psychology* 86, no. 2 (2011), 137–42.
8. Stephen G. Post, "Altruism, Happiness, and Health: It's Good to Be Good," *International Journal of Behavioral Medicine* 12, no. 2 (2005).
9. Lois Wladis Hoffman, *The Effects of the Mother's Employment on the Family and the Child*, 1998, lecture, Parenthood in America, March 20, 2014, http://parenthood.library.wisc.edu/Hoffman/Hoffman.html.
10. U.S. Census Bureau, *Decennial Censuses, 1890 to 1940, and Current Population Survey, Annual Social and Economic Supplements, 1947 to 2015* (Washington, DC: U.S. Department of Commerce, September 2015).

11. Wendy Wang and Kim Parker, *Record Share of Americans Have Never Married: As Values, Economics and Gender Patterns Change* (Washington, DC: Pew Research Center's Social & Demographic Trends project, September 2014).

12. Kay Hymowitz, Jason S. Carroll, W. Bradford Wilcox, and Kelleen Kaye, *Knot Yet: The Benefits and Costs of Delayed Marriage in America* (Washington, DC: The National Campaign to Prevent Teen and Unplanned Pregnancy, 2013).

13. Ibid.

14. Ibid.

15. Ibid.

16. Betsey Stevenson and Justin Wolfers, "Marriage and Divorce: Changes and their Driving Forces," *Journal of Economic Perspectives, American Economic Association* 21, no. 2 (Spring 2007), 27–52.

17. Ibid.

18. Wang and Parker, *Record Share of Americans Have Never Married.*

19. Arlie Russell Hochschild and Anne Machung, *The Second Shift* (New York: Penguin Books, 2003).

20. Hymowitz, Carroll, Wilcox, and Kaye, *Knot Yet.*

21. Centers for Disease Control and Prevention, *National Public Health Action Plan for the Detection, Prevention, and Management of Infertility* (Atlanta, GA: Centers for Disease Control and Prevention, June 2014).

22. American Society for Reproductive Medicine, "Quick Facts about Infertility," accessed June 11, 2012, http://www.asrm.org/detail.aspx?id=2322.

23. Amy Muise, Ulrich Schimmack, and Emily A. Impett, "Sexual Frequency Predicts Greater Well-Being, but More Is Not Always Better," *Social Psychological and Personality Science* 7 (May 2016), 295–302.

24. Daniel J. Kruger and Susan M. Hughes, "Tendencies to Fall Asleep First after Sex Are Associated with Greater Partner Desires for Bonding and Affection," *Journal of Social, Evolutionary, and Cultural Psychology* 5, no. 4 (2011), 239–247.

25. Stuart Brody, "The Relative Health Benefits of Different Sexual Activities," *Journal of Sexual Medicine* 7 (April 2010), 1336–1361.

26. NORC, *General Social Survey Final Report: Trends in Psychological Well-Being, 1972-2014* (Chicago: University of Chicago, 2015).

About the Authors

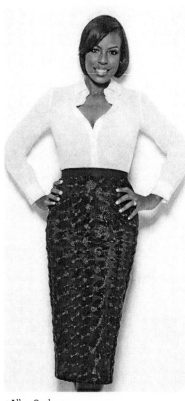

©Allen Cooley

Dion Metzger, MD is a board certified psychiatrist whose approachable demeanor and compelling expertise in mental health issues have helped her provide life-changing techniques that transform the lives of her patients.

It was during a psychology class her senior year in high school that Dr. Metzger developed an interest in human behavior. That led the New York native to Atlanta, Georgia, where she enrolled in Emory University and graduated with a bachelor's degree in Psychology. She earned her Doctorate of Medicine from Morehouse School of Medicine and completed her psychiatry residency at Emory University School of Medicine. In addition to obtaining her degrees, she also completed medical research at Stanford University School of Medicine and Centers for Disease Control and Prevention (CDC).

Dr. Metzger has used her deep well of experience in psychiatry to provide expertise through features on talk shows, in magazines, and in blogs discussing relationships, sex, jobs, and pop-culture behavioral health topics. She can be reached at www.dionmetzgermd.com.

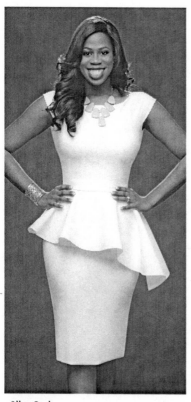

©Allen Cooley

Ayo Afejuku Gathing, MD is not only a board certified child, adolescent, and adult psychiatrist; she is a humanitarian, wife, loving family member, and friend to many. Dr. Gathing specializes in building healthy relationships and families, innovative health solutions, and the treatment of mental illness. As a professor, author, and dynamic speaker, she inspires others while imparting her knowledge of medicine with strategies for maintaining wellness.

Dr. Gathing obtained a Bachelor of Science in Applied Biology from the Georgia Institute of Technology, where she graduated with honors. She completed her psychiatric training and fellowship at the Emory University School of Medicine, where she received numerous awards and accolades and was nominated as the chief resident after graduating with a Medical Doctorate from the Morehouse School of Medicine. She sits on the Behavioral Health Advisory Committee for the State of Texas legislature and serves as a medical director in health-care administration, where she oversees the appropriate delivery of mental health services to indigent and special needs populations.

Dr. Gathing brings her expertise in the field of psychiatry to the masses through practical discussions and relatable delivery of health information. She is passionate in bringing a psychological perspective to modern concepts, such as relationships, parenting, career planning, and use of technology. She can be reached at www.ayogathingmd.com.